Difficult Conversations in Nursing & Healthcare: A Practical Guide to Speaking Up with Confidence and Compassion

Difficult Conversations, Volume 1

Rachael Benson

Published by Rachael Benson, 2025.

DIFFICULT CONVERSATIONS IN NURSING & HEALTHCARE: A PRACTICAL GUIDE TO SPEAKING UP WITH CONFIDENCE AND COMPASSION

First edition. August 23, 2025.

ISBN: 979-8232230876

Written by Rachael Benson.

Book Title: Difficult Conversations in Nursing & Healthcare: A Practical Guide to Speaking Up with Confidence and Compassion

Author: Rachael Benson

Book Description

In healthcare, silence can be costly. From safeguarding concerns and end-of-life care to workplace bullying and systemic bias, nurses, midwives, and health visitors face emotionally charged conversations every day. Yet many feel underprepared, unsupported, or afraid to speak up.

This essential guide empowers professionals to navigate difficult conversations with clarity, empathy, and courage. Drawing on real-world scenarios, evidence-based frameworks, and reflective practice, it offers practical tools for addressing emotional distress, advocating for patients, challenging unsafe practices, and fostering inclusive team cultures.

Whether you're newly qualified or a seasoned practitioner, this book will help you build confidence, protect wellbeing, and lead with integrity—because when nurses speak up, care improves.

Introduction

Why Difficult Conversations Matter in Nursing

Nursing is a profession built on compassion, skill, and communication. Yet, some of the most critical moments in a nurse's career are also the most challenging to navigate—those conversations that feel uncomfortable, emotionally charged, or ethically complex. Whether it's telling a family that their loved one is dying, confronting a colleague about unsafe practice, or addressing racism in the workplace, these moments require courage, clarity, and care.

Research and lived experience show that many nurses, midwives, and health visitors feel underprepared for these conversations. The consequences of avoidance can be profound: patient harm, team dysfunction, moral injury, and burnout. This book is designed to change that.

Difficult Conversations in Nursing offers practical strategies, real-world scenarios, and evidence-based frameworks to help you speak up with confidence and compassion. It is not just a guide—it's a toolkit for professional growth, patient advocacy, and personal resilience.

Whether you're a newly qualified nurse or a seasoned practitioner, this book will support you in navigating the conversations that matter most. Because when nurses speak up, care improves—and so do outcomes for everyone involved.

The Emotional and Professional Cost of Avoidance

Avoiding difficult conversations in healthcare settings—whether in hospitals, community clinics, or home visits—can have far-reaching consequences for nurses, health visitors, and midwives. While the instinct to preserve harmony or avoid conflict is understandable, silence often leads to deeper emotional strain and professional risk.

Emotional Toll

In both hospital and community settings, nurses work in close proximity to colleagues, often under intense pressure. When inappropriate behaviour, unsafe practices, or discriminatory language go unaddressed, it can leave staff feeling isolated, anxious, and morally compromised. Health visitors, who often work alone in homes or community spaces, may feel particularly vulnerable when faced with uncomfortable dynamics or safeguarding concerns. The emotional burden of witnessing but not addressing these issues can lead to moral distress—a condition where professionals feel unable to act according to their ethical beliefs.

Unresolved issues such as exclusion from team activities, inappropriate touching, or unprofessional conduct can leave nurses feeling threatened or undervalued. Over time, this erodes self-confidence, contributes to burnout, and diminishes job satisfaction. Nurses may begin to question their own professionalism or feel complicit in a culture that tolerates poor behaviour.

Professional Consequences

Avoidance also undermines the standards of care and accountability expected in nursing practice. In hospitals, failing to address concerns about medication errors, safety-critical incidents, or poor communication can directly impact patient outcomes. In community roles, such as health visiting, avoiding conversations about safeguarding, neglect, or cultural misunderstandings can delay vital interventions and compromise family support.

Professionally, avoidance can lead to:

- **Escalation of conflict**: Issues left unspoken often worsen over time, making resolution more difficult.
- **Breakdown of trust**: Colleagues may lose faith in each other's integrity or reliability.
- **Missed learning opportunities**: Constructive feedback is essential for growth and improvement.
- **Compromised patient safety**: Unchallenged errors or unsafe practices can have serious consequences.

Preparation, documentation, and emotional regulation when approaching difficult conversations is essential; delays in addressing issues can result in grievances, strained relationships, and systemic failures. Nurses are encouraged to reflect on power dynamics, seek support from managers or Human Resources, and use structured communication strategies to navigate these challenges.

A Culture of Courage

Ultimately, avoiding difficult conversations is not a neutral act—it is a decision that can perpetuate harm. Nurses, midwives, and health visitors must be equipped with the tools and confidence to speak up, not only for their own well-being but for the safety and dignity of those they care for. Creating a culture where difficult conversations are welcomed, supported, and resolved constructively is essential for a thriving healthcare system.

Why Difficult Conversations Are a Professional Imperative

In nursing, silence is rarely neutral. Avoiding difficult conversations doesn't just affect individual well-being—it can compromise the integrity of the entire healthcare system. Whether in hospitals, community clinics, or home visits, nurses, midwives, and health visitors are expected to uphold professional standards, advocate for patients, and contribute to safe, inclusive care environments. This requires speaking up, even when it's uncomfortable.

The Nursing and Midwifery Council (NMC) Code outlines a duty to act when concerns arise. Yet many nurses hesitate, fearing conflict, retaliation, or being misunderstood; preparation, emotional regulation, and professional boundaries are imperative. It reminds us that difficult conversations are not just interpersonal—they are clinical, ethical, and organisational.

In hospital settings, unresolved issues can lead to medication errors, breakdowns in communication, and unsafe practices. In community roles, avoidance may delay safeguarding interventions or perpetuate cultural misunderstandings. Health Visitors, often working independently, may feel particularly isolated when faced with sensitive concerns about parenting, neglect, or domestic abuse.

Avoidance also reinforces power imbalances. When junior staff feel unable to challenge senior colleagues, or when discriminatory behaviour goes unchecked, it sends a message that some voices matter more than others. This undermines psychological safety and discourages open dialogue—both of which are essential for effective teamwork and patient care.

Difficult conversations are not a disruption to nursing—they are part of it. They are how we uphold standards, protect patients, and support each other. This book is designed to help you approach these moments with confidence, compassion, and clarity—because when nurses speak up, the whole system becomes stronger.

How This Book Will Help

This book is designed to be a practical, compassionate, and empowering guide for nurses, midwives, and health visitors who face difficult conversations in their daily practice. Whether you're working in a busy hospital ward, visiting families in the community, or supporting patients through life-changing events, the ability to communicate clearly and courageously is essential.

You will find:

- **Evidence-based frameworks** for structuring sensitive conversations
- **Real-life scenarios** from diverse healthcare settings
- **Scripts and toolkits** to help you speak up with confidence
- **Reflective prompts** to support emotional resilience and professional growth

Each chapter is grounded in the realities of nursing practice, informed by research, and shaped by the voices of healthcare professionals. You'll learn how to navigate conversations about emotional distress, end-of-life care, unsafe practices, racism, and team dynamics—without losing compassion or professionalism.

Difficult conversations are not a sign of failure—they are a sign of leadership. They are how we protect patients, support colleagues, and uphold the values of our profession. This book will help you do just that.

For practical guidance, see Appendix 1: Difficult Conversations in Nursing: Toolkit

Part I: Conversations with Patients and Families

Chapter 1: Understanding Emotional Distress

"*People will forget what you said, people will forget what you did, but people will never forget how you made them feel.*"

— Maya Angelou

Emotional distress is a frequent companion to illness, injury, and uncertainty. In healthcare settings, nurses are often the first to witness and respond to the emotional needs of patients and their families. Whether it's the quiet anxiety of a patient awaiting test results, the grief of a family receiving bad news, or the frustration of someone navigating a long-term condition, these moments call for more than clinical skill—they require emotional presence and compassionate communication.

Yet many nurses feel unprepared for these conversations. The pressure to "stay professional," the fear of saying the wrong thing, and the emotional toll of repeated exposure to suffering can lead to avoidance or detachment. In busy hospital wards and community visits, time constraints and workload demand often leave little room for deep emotional engagement. But when emotional distress is overlooked or mishandled, it can affect not only the patient's experience but also the nurse's own sense of fulfilment and professional integrity.

This chapter explores how to recognise emotional distress, respond with empathy, and engage in conversations that support healing and trust. It introduces practical frameworks and strategies that help nurses navigate these moments with confidence and care—because acknowledging emotional pain is not a distraction from clinical work; it is part of it.

Recognising Emotional Distress

Emotional distress in patients and families can manifest in many ways—some obvious, others subtle. Nurses, midwives, and health visitors are often the first to notice these signs, whether in a hospital bed, a clinic waiting room, or a family's living room. Recognising emotional distress is the first step toward meaningful, compassionate communication.

Verbal and Non-Verbal Cues

Patients may express distress through words, but just as often, it's revealed in what they don't say. Common verbal indicators include:

- Expressions of fear, hopelessness, or confusion
- Repeated questions or requests for reassurance
- Statements like "I don't know how much more I can take" or "I feel like a burden"

Non-verbal cues can be just as telling:

- Tearfulness or visible agitation
- Withdrawal, silence, or avoidance of eye contact
- Changes in posture, tone, or energy levels

Families may show distress through overprotectiveness, anger, or emotional detachment. Health visitors may notice signs of distress in parents who appear overwhelmed, disengaged, or excessively anxious about their child's development.

Cultural and Individual Differences

It's important to remember that emotional distress is shaped by culture, personality, and life experience. Some patients may openly express their emotions, while others may suppress them due to cultural norms or fear of stigma. Nurses must approach each individual with sensitivity, avoiding assumptions and remaining open to different expressions of pain.

For example:

- In some cultures, stoicism is valued, and emotional expression may be seen as weakness.
- In others, emotional openness is encouraged, and distress may be shared freely.

Understanding these differences helps nurses avoid misinterpretation and respond appropriately.

The Importance of Attunement

Recognising emotional distress isn't just about observation—it's about attunement. This means being emotionally present, noticing subtle shifts in mood or behaviour, and responding with empathy. It requires slowing down, even briefly, to connect with the human experience behind the clinical presentation.

In busy healthcare environments, this can be challenging. But even a few moments of genuine connection can make a profound difference in how a patient feels—and how a nurse feels about their work.

The Role of the Nurse

Nurses occupy a unique position in the healthcare system—not only as clinical professionals but also as emotional anchors for patients and families. Whether in a hospital ward, a community clinic, or a family home, nurses are often the most consistent point of contact. This proximity means they are frequently the first to notice emotional distress and the most trusted to respond.

Being Present and Emotionally Attuned

The role of the nurse in emotionally charged situations is not to fix or solve, but to be present. Emotional attunement involves noticing subtle cues, listening deeply, and responding with empathy. It's about creating a space where patients feel seen and heard, even when their distress cannot be immediately resolved.

This presence is especially important in community and health visiting roles, where patients may be isolated or navigating complex social challenges. A nurse's ability to offer calm, compassionate attention can be a lifeline.

Balancing Empathy with Professional Boundaries

While empathy is essential, nurses must also maintain professional boundaries. Emotional involvement must be balanced with clinical objectivity to avoid burnout and ensure safe care.

This means:

- Recognising when emotional support becomes therapeutic and requires referral
- Avoiding over-identification with patients' experiences
- Using supervision and reflective practice to process emotional encounters

Boundaries are not barriers—they are tools that allow nurses to care effectively without becoming overwhelmed.

Listening Without Fixing

One of the most powerful roles a nurse can play is that of a listener. Patients in distress often need to express their fears, frustrations, or grief without being interrupted or "fixed."

Nurses can support this by:

- Allowing silence
- Reflecting back what they hear
- Validating emotions without rushing to reassure or redirect

This kind of listening builds trust and helps patients feel emotionally safe, which is essential for healing and cooperation.

Advocacy and Emotional Safety

Nurses also play a critical role in advocating for patients' emotional needs within the wider healthcare team. This includes:

- Raising concerns when emotional distress is overlooked
- Ensuring patients have access to psychological support
- Challenging practices that may cause emotional harm

In doing so, nurses help create a culture of emotional safety—one where patients and staff alike feel respected, supported, and valued.

Communication Frameworks

Effective communication is at the heart of nursing practice, especially when responding to emotional distress. While empathy and intuition are vital, structured frameworks can help nurses feel more confident and consistent in their approach. These tools provide a roadmap for navigating sensitive conversations with clarity, compassion, and professionalism.

The NURSE Framework

The NURSE acronym is a widely used model for responding to emotional cues in clinical settings. It helps nurses validate emotions and build rapport without overwhelming the patient or losing focus.

- Name the emotion: "It sounds like you're feeling overwhelmed."
- Understand: "I can see why this situation would be upsetting."
- Respect: "You've been incredibly strong through all of this."
- Support: "I'm here to help however I can."
- Explore: "Can you tell me more about what's been hardest for you?"

This framework encourages emotional presence while maintaining professional boundaries. It's particularly useful in moments of grief, fear, or frustration, and can be adapted for use with families and carers.

Active Listening and Reflective Responses

Active listening involves more than hearing—it requires full attention, empathy, and thoughtful responses. Key techniques include:

- **Paraphrasing**: "So what I'm hearing is that you're feeling anxious about the next steps."
- **Reflecting feelings**: "It sounds like this has been really difficult for you."
- **Clarifying**: "Can I check that I've understood you correctly?"

These responses help patients feel heard and understood, which can reduce distress and build trust.

Using Silence and Body Language

Silence can be a powerful tool in emotionally charged conversations. Allowing space for patients to process their thoughts or emotions shows respect and patience. Nurses should also be mindful of:

- **Body posture**: Open and relaxed
- **Facial expressions**: Calm and attentive
- **Eye contact**: Gentle and appropriate

Non-verbal communication often speaks louder than words. A nurse's presence—calm, grounded, and attentive—can offer comfort even when words are hard to find.

Adapting Frameworks to Context

While frameworks are helpful, they must be adapted to the individual and the situation. For example:

- In a hospital setting, time may be limited, so brief but meaningful responses are key.
- In community visits, there may be more space for extended dialogue and exploration.
- With families, especially in safeguarding or end-of-life contexts, sensitivity and clarity are essential.

The goal is not to follow a script, but to use these tools to guide compassionate, confident communication.

Practical Strategies

Recognising emotional distress is only the first step—knowing how to respond is what transforms awareness into compassionate care. This section offers practical strategies for initiating and navigating emotionally sensitive conversations with patients and families, whether in hospital, community, or home settings.

Starting the Conversation

Opening a dialogue about emotional distress can feel daunting, especially when time is limited or emotions are high. Here are some gentle, non-intrusive ways to begin:

- "You seem a bit quieter today—how are you feeling?"
- "It's completely understandable to feel overwhelmed. Would you like to talk about it?"
- "I'm here to listen if there's anything on your mind."

These openers invite conversation without pressure, signalling empathy and availability.

Validating Without Overwhelming

Validation helps patients feel seen and heard. It's important to acknowledge emotions without trying to fix them immediately:

- "It makes sense that you're feeling anxious—this is a lot to take in."
- "You've been through so much. It's okay to feel upset."
- "That sounds incredibly difficult. Thank you for sharing it with me."

Avoid phrases that dismiss or minimise distress, such as "Don't worry," "Stay positive," or "Others have it worse." These can unintentionally shut down emotional expression.

Managing Emotional Reactions

Patients may cry, become angry, withdraw, or express frustration. Nurses can respond by:

- Remaining calm and grounded
- Offering tissues or a quiet space
- Using reflective statements: "It sounds like this has been building up for a while."

If emotions escalate, it's okay to pause and suggest a follow-up conversation. Emotional safety is just as important as physical safety.

Adapting to Context

- **In hospitals**: Time may be limited, so brief but meaningful exchanges matter. Even a few minutes of focused attention can make a difference.
- **In community settings**: Nurses may have more time and privacy, allowing for deeper conversations and follow-up.
- **With families**: Sensitivity is key, especially when discussing prognosis, safeguarding, or long-term care.

Using Support Systems

If a conversation reveals deeper emotional needs, nurses should:

- Refer to psychological services or pastoral care
- Document concerns clearly and factually
- Discuss the situation in supervision or team meetings

Knowing when to escalate or seek support is part of professional responsibility.

Case Study: "I Just Don't Know What to Do Anymore"

Scenario

During a routine community visit, a nurse meets with Mr. A, a 68-year-old man recently diagnosed with heart failure. He lives alone and has been struggling to manage his medication and diet. As the nurse begins the visit, Mr. A sighs deeply and says, "I just don't know what to do anymore."

His tone is flat, his posture slumped. He avoids eye contact and seems withdrawn. The nurse senses emotional distress but is unsure whether to explore it or focus on the clinical checklist.

Response Using the NURSE Framework

Instead of moving straight into clinical tasks, the nurse gently responds:

- **Name**: "It sounds like you're feeling overwhelmed."
- **Understand**: "Managing everything on your own must be really tough."
- **Respect**: "You've been doing your best to stay on top of things, and that takes strength."
- **Support**: "I'm here to help. We can look at what's working and what's not."
- **Explore**: "Can you tell me more about what's been hardest lately?"

Mr. A begins to open up. He shares that he's been feeling isolated and unsure about his future. He's worried about being a burden to his family and feels ashamed for not coping better.

Outcome and Reflection

By responding with empathy and structure, the nurse creates a safe space for Mr. A to express his emotions. Together, they identify practical steps—adjusting his medication schedule, arranging a follow-up with his GP, and connecting him with a local support group.

The nurse documents the conversation factually and discusses it in supervision to reflect on the emotional impact and ensure continuity of care.

Key Learning Points

- Emotional distress often surfaces in subtle ways—listen for cues.
- Structured frameworks like NURSE help guide compassionate responses.
- Emotional support is part of holistic care, not separate from it.
- Reflective practice helps nurses process and learn from these encounters.

Challenges and Barriers

- Despite the importance of addressing emotional distress, nurses often face significant challenges that make these conversations difficult to initiate or sustain. These barriers are not just personal—they are systemic, cultural, and organisational.

Time Pressures and Workload

- In both hospital and community settings, nurses are under constant pressure to manage clinical tasks, documentation, and patient flow. Emotional conversations can feel like a luxury in environments where every minute counts. This can lead to rushed interactions, missed cues, or avoidance of deeper engagement.

- Yet, delaying these conversations can allow distress to escalate. Even brief, well-timed interventions can make a meaningful difference.

Fear of Saying the Wrong Thing

- Many nurses worry about making things worse by saying the wrong thing. This fear can lead to silence or overly clinical responses that miss the emotional core of the issue. Without training or support, nurses may feel ill-equipped to handle grief, trauma, or existential distress.
- This is especially true in community roles, where nurses may be alone with patients and families, without immediate access to colleagues or supervisors for guidance.

Emotional Fatigue and Burnout

- Repeated exposure to suffering, loss, and complex social issues can take a toll. Nurses may begin to emotionally withdraw as a coping mechanism, leading to reduced empathy and increased detachment. This is not a failure—it's a sign of emotional overload.
- Supervision, reflective practice, and peer support are essential tools for managing this fatigue and maintaining emotional resilience.

Cultural and Organisational Norms

- In some healthcare environments, emotional conversations are discouraged or undervalued. A culture of "just get on with it" can prevent nurses from expressing concern or

seeking support. Hierarchical structures may also make it difficult to challenge senior colleagues or raise sensitive issues.
- Health visitors and community nurses may face additional challenges when navigating family dynamics, safeguarding concerns, or cultural misunderstandings—all of which require careful, confident communication.

Lack of Training and Confidence

- Many nurses report that they received little formal training in communication skills related to emotional distress. Without frameworks or practice, even experienced professionals may feel unsure about how to respond.
- This book aims to fill that gap—providing tools, language, and strategies to help nurses feel more confident and prepared.

Supporting Yourself

Engaging with emotional distress—especially on a regular basis—can be deeply rewarding, but also emotionally taxing. Nurses, midwives, and health visitors often carry the weight of others' pain while managing their own professional responsibilities. To sustain compassionate care, it's essential to prioritise your own emotional wellbeing.

Emotional Resilience

Resilience isn't about being unaffected by distress—it's about recovering and adapting. Building emotional resilience involves:

- **Recognising your limits**: Knowing when you're emotionally depleted and need rest or support.
- **Practising self-compassion**: Acknowledging that you're

doing your best, even when outcomes are difficult.

- **Creating boundaries**: Separating work stress from personal life where possible.

Simple practices like deep breathing, journaling, or taking short breaks during shifts can help regulate emotional responses and prevent overwhelm.

Supervision and Reflective Practice

Supervision—whether clinical, managerial, or reflective—is a vital space for processing emotional experiences. It allows nurses to:

- Talk through challenging conversations
- Receive feedback and validation
- Explore emotional reactions and ethical dilemmas

Reflective practice, such as writing in a journal or using structured models like Gibbs or Schön, helps nurses learn from experience and maintain emotional clarity.

"Reflection is not a luxury—it's a necessity for safe, ethical, and sustainable practice."

Debriefing and Peer Support

After emotionally intense conversations, debriefing with a trusted colleague or supervisor can help release tension and gain perspective. Peer support groups, informal chats, or structured team debriefs can foster connection and reduce isolation.

Health visitors and community nurses, who often work alone, may benefit from scheduled peer check-ins or virtual supervision sessions to stay emotionally supported.

Knowing When to Seek Help

If emotional distress begins to affect your sleep, mood, relationships, or ability to work, it's important to seek professional support. This may include:

- Occupational health services
- Counselling or therapy
- Speaking with a line manager or union representative

Seeking help is not a weakness—it's a professional strength. It ensures you can continue to care for others without compromising your own wellbeing.

SUMMARY OF KEY POINTS

- Emotional distress is common in healthcare and often expressed subtly.
- Nurses play a vital role in recognising and responding to emotional needs.
- Frameworks like NURSE and active listening techniques support compassionate communication.
- Practical strategies—such as validating emotions, managing reactions, and adapting to context—help nurses engage effectively.
- Challenges like time pressure, emotional fatigue, and lack of training can hinder these conversations.
- Supporting yourself through supervision, reflection, and peer support is essential for sustainable practice.

For practical guidance see Appendix 2: Conversation Frameworks Toolkit

Conclusion

Emotional distress is a common yet often overlooked aspect of healthcare. Nurses, midwives, and health visitors are uniquely positioned to recognise and respond to these moments—not just with clinical skill, but with compassion and presence. By using structured communication frameworks, active listening, and reflective practice, professionals can support patients and families through some of their most vulnerable experiences.

Acknowledging emotional pain is not a distraction from care—it is part of it. When nurses respond with empathy and clarity, they not only ease suffering but strengthen trust, safety, and healing. Emotional conversations are not a sign of weakness—they are a sign of professional strength.

Chapter 2: End-of-Life and Existential Conversations

"To care for those who once cared for us is one of the highest honours."

— Tia Walker

Few conversations in nursing are as emotionally charged or ethically complex as those surrounding death, dying, and existential distress. Whether in a hospital ward, hospice, or community setting, nurses are often present at the most vulnerable moments in a person's life. These conversations are not only about clinical decisions—they are about meaning, identity, fear, and love.

Patients facing the end of life may grapple with profound questions: *What happens next? Have I lived well? Will I be remembered?* Families may struggle with anticipatory grief, guilt, or conflict over care decisions. Nurses, meanwhile, must balance compassion with clarity, and empathy with professional boundaries.

Despite the frequency of these encounters, many nurses feel unprepared. The discomfort of discussing death, the fear of causing distress, and the complexity of cultural and spiritual beliefs can lead to avoidance or overly clinical responses. Yet silence in these moments can leave patients and families feeling isolated, confused, or emotionally unsupported.

This chapter explores how to engage in end-of-life and existential conversations with sensitivity, confidence, and care. It introduces practical frameworks, ethical considerations, and real-world strategies to help nurses navigate these deeply human moments. Because when we speak honestly and listen deeply, we honour not only the patient's life—but their dignity in death.

Understanding Existential Distress

Existential distress refers to the deep emotional and psychological suffering that arises when individuals confront the fundamental questions of life—especially in the face of serious illness, loss, or impending death. Unlike clinical depression or anxiety, existential distress is rooted in a person's search for meaning, identity, and purpose.

What Is Existential Distress?

Patients experiencing existential distress may express:

- Fear of dying or the unknown
- Loss of control or autonomy
- Feelings of isolation or abandonment
- Questions about the meaning of their life or suffering
- Regret, guilt, or unfinished business

This distress can be subtle or overt. A patient might say, "What's the point of all this?" or "I'm not the person I used to be." Others may withdraw, become irritable, or express hopelessness.

Existential distress is not a diagnosis—it's a human experience. Nurses, often present during these vulnerable moments, play a vital role in recognising and responding to it with sensitivity and respect.

Cultural and Spiritual Dimensions

Existential distress is shaped by cultural, spiritual, and personal beliefs. For some, faith provides comfort and clarity; for others, it may raise questions or conflict. Nurses must approach these conversations with cultural humility, avoiding assumptions and remaining open to diverse worldviews.

Key considerations include:

- Respecting spiritual beliefs and rituals
- Understanding cultural norms around death and dying
- Supporting patients in expressing their values and fears

In community settings, health visitors and palliative care nurses may encounter families navigating these issues in the privacy of their homes, where cultural and relational dynamics are especially pronounced.

Why It Matters in Nursing

Existential distress can affect a patient's emotional wellbeing, decision-making, and engagement with care. If left unaddressed, it may lead to withdrawal, non-compliance, or emotional suffering. Nurses who recognise and respond to existential distress help patients feel seen—not just as bodies to be treated, but as people with stories, fears, and hopes.

Supporting existential distress doesn't require having all the answers. It requires presence, empathy, and the courage to sit with discomfort. Sometimes, the most healing response is simply: "I'm here with you."

The Nurse's Role in End-of-Life Care

Nurses are often the constant presence in a patient's final days—providing not only clinical care but emotional support, advocacy, and dignity. In hospitals, hospices, and community settings, nurses are uniquely positioned to guide patients and families through the complexities of dying with compassion and clarity.

Being Present and Emotionally Available

End-of-life care is not just about managing symptoms—it's about being present. Nurses offer comfort through their presence, listening, and gentle reassurance. This emotional availability helps patients feel less alone and more supported in facing their fears, regrets, and hopes.

Being present means:

- Sitting quietly with a patient who is afraid
- Holding space for families to express grief
- Responding to emotional cues with empathy, not avoidance

Even brief moments of connection can have a profound impact on how patients experience their final days.

Supporting Dignity, Autonomy, and Comfort

Nurses play a vital role in preserving dignity at the end of life. This includes:

- Respecting patients' wishes and values
- Facilitating choices around care, environment, and rituals
- Advocating for comfort and symptom control

In community settings, this may involve coordinating with family members, GPs, and palliative care teams to ensure the patient's preferences are honoured at home.

Advocating for Patient Wishes and Values

Patients nearing the end of life may struggle to express their wishes, especially if family members or professionals hold differing views. Nurses often act as mediators and advocates, ensuring that the patient's voice remains central.

This may involve:

- Clarifying advance care plans or DNACPR decisions
- Supporting patients in expressing their goals and fears
- Navigating ethical dilemmas with sensitivity and professionalism

Advocacy is not about taking sides—it's about ensuring that care aligns with the patient's values and dignity.

Emotional Intelligence and Ethical Awareness

End-of-life care requires emotional intelligence: the ability to recognise, understand, and respond to complex emotions in oneself and others. It also demands ethical awareness, especially when navigating decisions about disclosure, treatment withdrawal, or family conflict.

Nurses must balance empathy with clarity, and compassion with clinical responsibility. This is not easy—but it is essential.

Communication Frameworks for End-of-Life Conversations

End-of-life conversations are emotionally complex and often unpredictable. Patients and families may be overwhelmed, frightened, or in denial. Nurses need communication tools that offer structure, sensitivity, and clarity—especially when delivering difficult news or supporting decision-making.

The SPIKES Protocol

Originally developed for oncology settings, the SPIKES protocol is widely used for delivering bad news in healthcare. It provides a step-by-step guide for structuring emotionally sensitive conversations:

- **S – Setting**: Ensure privacy, sit down, and minimise interruptions.
- **P – Perception**: Assess what the patient or family already understands.
- **I – Invitation**: Ask how much detail they want to know.
- **K – Knowledge**: Share information clearly and compassionately.
- **E – Emotions**: Respond to emotional reactions with empathy.
- **S – Strategy and Summary**: Discuss next steps and provide support.

Example:

"I can see this is very difficult to hear. We'll take this one step at a time, and I'll be here to support you."

SPIKES helps nurses balance honesty with compassion, especially when discussing prognosis, treatment limitations, or transitions to palliative care.

The VALUE Model for Family Meetings

The VALUE model is designed to support families during end-of-life care discussions:

- **V – Value** what the family says
- **A – Acknowledge** emotions

- **L – Listen** actively
- **U – Understand** the patient as a person
- **E – Elicit** questions and concerns

This model encourages relational, person-centred dialogue and is especially useful in multidisciplinary meetings or hospice settings.

Open-Ended Questions and Silence

Sometimes, the most powerful communication tools are the simplest. Open-ended questions invite reflection and emotional expression:

- "What worries you most right now?"
- "What does a good day look like for you?"
- "Is there anything you'd like us to know about your values or wishes?"

Silence, when used intentionally, allows space for processing and emotion. Nurses should resist the urge to fill every pause—sometimes, presence is more powerful than words.

Adapting Frameworks to Context

These frameworks are not rigid scripts—they are guides. Nurses must adapt them to:

- The patient's cognitive and emotional state
- Cultural and spiritual beliefs
- The urgency and setting of the conversation

In community nursing and health visiting, conversations may unfold gradually over multiple visits. In hospital settings, they may occur in high-pressure moments. Flexibility, empathy, and preparation are key.

Practical Strategies

End-of-life conversations are rarely straightforward. Emotions run high, circumstances vary, and each patient and family bring their own beliefs, fears, and expectations. Nurses need practical, adaptable strategies to navigate these moments with confidence and compassion.

Talking About Prognosis and Dying

Patients may ask direct or indirect questions about their condition. Nurses can respond with honesty, empathy, and clarity:

- "Would you like to talk about what's ahead?"
- "I can share what we know so far, and we'll take it step by step."
- "It's okay to feel uncertain—this is a difficult time."

Avoid euphemisms that obscure reality. Phrases like "passing away" or "not doing well" can confuse or mislead. Instead, use clear but gentle language, tailored to the patient's readiness.

Responding to Difficult Questions

Patients may ask:

- "Am I going to die?"
- "How long do I have?"
- "What happens after?"

These questions require sensitivity. Nurses don't need to have all the answers—but they can offer presence and honesty:

- "That's a very important question. Let's talk about what we know and what we can plan together."
- "I don't have a definite answer, but I'll be here with you through it."

If spiritual or existential questions arise, nurses can support exploration or refer to chaplaincy or psychological services.

Supporting Families Through Grief and Decision-Making

Families may struggle with anticipatory grief, guilt, or conflict. Nurses can help by:

- Facilitating open conversations: "What are your hopes and concerns for your loved one?"
- Clarifying care plans and options
- Encouraging shared decision-making and emotional expression

In community settings, this may involve multiple visits and ongoing support. In hospital settings, it may require coordination with palliative care teams and family meetings.

Managing Emotional Reactions

Patients and families may cry, become angry, or withdraw. Nurses can respond by:

- Remaining calm and grounded
- Validating emotions: "It's okay to feel this way."
- Offering space and time: "Would you like a moment alone or someone to talk to?"

If emotions escalate, nurses should use de-escalation techniques and consider involving senior staff or support services.

Adapting to Context and Culture

End-of-life conversations must be adapted to:

- Cultural beliefs about death and dying
- Language and literacy levels
- Family dynamics and decision-making roles

Nurses should approach each situation with cultural humility, asking open questions and respecting diverse practices.

Case Study: "She Doesn't Know Yet"

Scenario

During a hospital shift, a nurse is caring for Mrs. L, a 72-year-old woman recently diagnosed with advanced pancreatic cancer. The medical team has discussed the prognosis with her family, who have requested that the nurse not tell Mrs. L about the seriousness of her condition. "She doesn't know yet," her daughter says. "We don't want her to give up."

The nurse is caught in a difficult position—balancing the family's wishes, the patient's right to know, and her own ethical responsibilities.

Ethical and Emotional Considerations

This situation raises several ethical questions:

- Does Mrs. L have the right to know her diagnosis and prognosis?
- Is withholding information protecting her—or denying her autonomy?
- How can the nurse support the family's emotional needs while advocating for the patient?

Emotionally, the nurse feels conflicted. She wants to respect the family's grief and protect Mrs. L from distress, but she also senses that Mrs. L suspects something is wrong. The nurse notices Mrs. L asking vague questions like, "Is this serious?" and "Why do I feel so tired all the time?"

Navigating the Conversation

The nurse decides to approach the situation with sensitivity and structure. She uses elements of the SPIKES protocol to guide her response:

- She ensures privacy and a calm setting.
- She gently explores Mrs. L's understanding: "What have the doctors shared with you so far?"
- She listens carefully to Mrs. L's concerns and emotional cues.
- She avoids giving false reassurance, instead offering support: "It's okay to have questions. I'm here to talk through anything you'd like to know."

The nurse also speaks with the medical team and palliative care service to ensure a coordinated approach. Together, they plan a family meeting to discuss how best to support Mrs. L with honesty and compassion.

Outcome and Reflection

Mrs. L is eventually informed of her diagnosis in a sensitive, supportive conversation involving her consultant and nurse. She expresses relief at knowing the truth and begins to make decisions about her care and legacy. The family, though initially hesitant, appreciates the transparency and feels better equipped to support her.

The nurse reflects on the importance of:

- Advocating for patient autonomy
- Using structured communication tools
- Seeking support from colleagues and supervisors

This case illustrates the complexity of end-of-life conversations and the vital role nurses play in navigating them with empathy, ethics, and professionalism.

Barriers and Challenges

End-of-life and existential conversations are among the most emotionally and ethically demanding in nursing practice. Despite their importance, nurses often encounter significant barriers that make these conversations difficult to initiate or sustain.

Time Constraints and Clinical Pressures

In acute hospital settings, nurses may be responsible for multiple patients with complex needs. The urgency of clinical tasks—medication rounds, documentation, and responding to deteriorating conditions—can leave little time for meaningful emotional engagement. In community settings, health visitors and district nurses may face tight schedules and lone working conditions that limit opportunities for extended dialogue.

Yet, avoiding these conversations due to time pressure can lead to missed opportunities for emotional support, advance care planning, and patient-centred decision-making.

Fear of Causing Distress or Saying the Wrong Thing

Many nurses worry that discussing death or prognosis will upset patients or families, or that they'll say something inappropriate. This fear can lead to avoidance, vague language, or deferring the conversation to doctors. While well-intentioned, this can leave patients feeling confused, isolated, or excluded from decisions about their own care.

Training in communication frameworks and emotional literacy can help nurses feel more confident and prepared.

Cultural and Family Dynamics

Cultural beliefs about death, disclosure, and decision-making vary widely. In some cultures, families may request that patients not be told the full truth about their condition. In others, spiritual or religious practices may shape how end-of-life care is approached.

Nurses must navigate these dynamics with cultural humility—respecting beliefs while advocating for patient autonomy and ethical transparency.

Ethical Dilemmas and Role Boundaries

Nurses may face ethical tension between respecting family wishes and upholding the patient's right to know. They may feel caught between medical decisions made by doctors and the emotional needs of patients. In some cases, nurses may be excluded from key conversations, despite being the most consistent presence in the patient's care.

Clear policies, team communication, and access to ethics support can help nurses navigate these dilemmas.

Emotional Impact and Burnout

Repeated exposure to death, grief, and existential suffering can take a toll. Nurses may experience compassion fatigue, moral distress, or emotional exhaustion. Without adequate support, this can lead to withdrawal, cynicism, or burnout.

Supervision, reflective practice, and peer support are essential for sustaining emotional resilience and professional integrity.

Supporting Yourself in End-of-Life Work

Caring for patients at the end of life is one of the most profound responsibilities in nursing. It can also be one of the most emotionally demanding. Nurses often absorb the grief, fear, and existential pain of others while managing their own emotional responses. Without adequate support, this can lead to compassion fatigue, burnout, or moral distress.

Acknowledging the Emotional Impact

End-of-life care is not just clinically complex—it's emotionally intense. Nurses may experience:

- Grief after a patient's death
- Guilt over decisions or outcomes
- Emotional exhaustion from repeated exposure to suffering

Acknowledging these feelings is the first step toward processing them. Suppressing emotions may seem like a way to stay professional, but over time, it can lead to detachment or burnout.

Using Supervision and Reflective Practice

Supervision—whether clinical, managerial, or reflective—is essential for emotional wellbeing. It provides a safe space to:

- Talk through difficult conversations
- Explore ethical dilemmas
- Receive validation and guidance

Reflective practice helps nurses make sense of their experiences. Journaling, peer discussions, or using models like Gibbs or Schön can support emotional clarity and professional growth.

"Reflection turns experience into insight."

Creating Emotional Boundaries

Boundaries are not barriers—they are safeguards. Nurses must learn to:

- Separate their personal emotions from professional responsibilities
- Recognise when they are becoming emotionally overwhelmed
- Step back when needed, without guilt

This is especially important in community and palliative care settings, where relationships with patients and families may be long-term and deeply personal.

Building Resilience Through Meaning-Making

Finding meaning in end-of-life work can be a powerful source of resilience. Nurses often describe this work as a privilege—being present at the end of someone's life, offering comfort, and preserving dignity.

Strategies for meaning making include:

- Reflecting on the impact of your care
- Celebrating small moments of connection
- Sharing stories with colleagues

Seeking Support When Needed

If emotional distress begins to affect your sleep, mood, relationships, or ability to work, it's important to seek help. This may include:

- Occupational health services
- Counselling or therapy
- Speaking with a line manager or union representative

Seeking support is not a weakness—it's a professional strength. It ensures you can continue to care for others without compromising your own wellbeing.

Summary of Key Points

- **End-of-life and existential conversations** are emotionally and ethically complex but essential to compassionate care.
- Nurses play a **central role** in supporting patients and families through grief, uncertainty, and decision-making.
- Frameworks like **SPIKES** and **VALUE** provide structure for delivering difficult news and facilitating family dialogue.
- **Cultural humility**, emotional intelligence, and ethical awareness are critical in navigating diverse beliefs and dynamics.
- Avoidance can lead to **emotional isolation**, missed opportunities for planning, and compromised dignity.
- Nurses must also care for themselves—through **supervision**, **reflection**, and **peer support**—to sustain resilience and compassion.

For practical guidance see Appendix3: End of Life Conversations Toolkit

Closing Reflection

End-of-life conversations are not just about death—they are about life, meaning, and dignity. When nurses speak with honesty and compassion, they help patients and families find peace, clarity, and connection. These moments, though difficult, are among the most profound in nursing practice. With the right tools, support, and courage, you can navigate them with grace and integrity.

Conclusion

End-of-life and existential conversations are among the most profound and challenging moments in nursing practice. They require not only clinical clarity but emotional intelligence, cultural sensitivity, and ethical awareness. When nurses engage with patients and families during these vulnerable times—with honesty, empathy, and presence—they uphold dignity, foster trust, and support healing.

These conversations are not just about death—they are about life, meaning, and connection. By using structured frameworks, reflective practice, and compassionate communication, nurses can navigate these moments with grace and integrity. In doing so, they honour the humanity at the heart of healthcare.

Chapter 3: Navigating Consent, Capacity, and Risk

"Informed consent is not just a signature—it's a conversation."

In nursing practice, few conversations are as legally and ethically significant as those involving consent, capacity, and risk. Whether you're discussing treatment options with a patient, raising safeguarding concerns with a family, or assessing a young person's ability to make decisions, these moments demand clarity, sensitivity, and professional confidence.

Yet many nurses feel uncertain when navigating these topics. The Mental Capacity Act (2005), safeguarding legislation, and professional codes of conduct provide essential guidance—but applying them in real-world conversations can be challenging. Patients may be confused, distressed, or resistant. Families may disagree or feel overwhelmed. Nurses may worry about saying the wrong thing, breaching confidentiality, or escalating unnecessarily.

This chapter is designed to help you approach these conversations with confidence and care. You'll explore how to assess capacity, gain informed consent, and communicate risk in ways that uphold dignity, protect safety, and respect autonomy. You'll also learn how to work effectively with vulnerable adults, young people, and multidisciplinary teams—especially when safeguarding concerns arise.

Because when nurses speak clearly and compassionately about consent, capacity, and risk, they don't just follow the law—they protect lives, empower patients, and strengthen trust.

Legal and Ethical Considerations

Conversations about consent, capacity, and risk are not just clinical—they are legal and ethical imperatives. Nurses, midwives, and health visitors must navigate these discussions with clarity, compassion, and confidence, especially when working with vulnerable individuals or in safeguarding contexts. Understanding the legal frameworks and ethical principles that underpin these conversations is essential for safe, respectful, and accountable practice.

The Mental Capacity Act (2005)

The **Mental Capacity Act (MCA)** provides the legal foundation for decision-making with individuals aged 16 and over in England and Wales. It outlines five key principles:

1. **Presumption of capacity**: Every adult is assumed to have capacity unless proven otherwise.
2. **Support to make decisions**: All practical steps must be taken to help someone make their own decision.
3. **Right to make unwise decisions**: Making a decision others disagree with does not mean a person lacks capacity.
4. **Best interests**: If a person lacks capacity, decisions must be made in their best interests.
5. **Least restrictive option**: Any intervention must be the least restrictive of the person's rights and freedoms.

Capacity assessments must be **decision-specific** and **time-specific**. Nurses must determine whether the person can:

- Understand relevant information,

- Retain it long enough to make a decision,
- Use or weigh it as part of the decision-making process,
- Communicate their decision (verbally, non-verbally, or otherwise).

In practice, this means documenting clearly, involving family or advocates when appropriate, and seeking support from senior staff or safeguarding leads when capacity is in doubt.

Informed Consent

Consent is valid only when it is:

- **Voluntary**: Given freely, without pressure or coercion.
- **Informed**: Based on clear, understandable information.
- **Capacitated**: Given by someone with the mental ability to decide.

Nurses must ensure patients understand the nature, purpose, risks, and alternatives of any proposed intervention. This includes:

- Using plain language,
- Checking understanding,
- Adapting communication for cognitive, cultural, or language barriers.

In community settings, health visitors may need to explain consent for developmental assessments, safeguarding referrals, or home safety checks—often in emotionally sensitive contexts. In hospital settings, time pressures must not compromise the quality of consent conversations.

Safeguarding and Risk

Nurses have a **legal duty to safeguard** children and adults at risk of harm. This includes:

- Recognising signs of abuse, neglect, or exploitation,
- Raising concerns through appropriate safeguarding channels,
- Communicating risk clearly and compassionately.

Safeguarding conversations can be difficult. Families may feel judged or defensive. Patients may be reluctant to disclose abuse or may lack capacity to protect themselves. Nurses must balance empathy with professional responsibility, using structured tools (e.g., SBAR) and seeking support from safeguarding leads or multidisciplinary teams.

Ethical Principles in Practice

Legal frameworks guide action, but **ethical principles** shape how those actions are carried out. Key principles include:

- **Autonomy**: Respecting the individual's right to make decisions.
- **Beneficence**: Acting in the person's best interests.
- **Non-maleficence**: Avoiding harm.
- **Justice**: Ensuring fairness and equity.

Ethical dilemmas often arise when these principles conflict—for example, when a patient refuses treatment that could save their life, or when a family wants to withhold information from a dying relative. Nurses must reflect, consult, and document carefully, using supervision and ethics support when needed.

Case Study: "She Said Yes, But I'm Not Sure She Understood"

Scenario

During a busy afternoon shift in a hospital ward, Nurse J is asked to obtain consent from Mrs. K, a 78-year-old woman with early-stage dementia, for a CT scan. Mrs. K appears cooperative and nods when asked if she agrees to the procedure. However, Nurse J notices that Mrs. K seems confused about why the scan is needed and repeatedly asks, "Will this make me better?"

Nurse J feels uneasy. The doctor is waiting, the radiology slot is booked, and Mrs. K has technically "consented." But has she truly understood? Is her capacity to consent intact? Nurse J wonders whether to delay the scan, escalate the concern, or proceed as planned.

Reflection

This scenario highlights the tension between clinical efficiency and ethical responsibility. It raises key questions:

- How do we assess capacity in time-pressured environments?
- What does "informed" consent really mean?
- When should nurses speak up—and how?

Learning Points

- Consent is not valid unless the patient has capacity and understands the information.
- The Mental Capacity Act (2005) provides a framework for assessing decision-making ability.
- Nurses have a duty to advocate for patients when capacity is unclear or consent feels coerced.
- Speaking up may feel disruptive—but it protects patient rights and professional integrity.

Communicating Risk and Safeguarding Concerns

Safeguarding conversations are among the most sensitive and complex that nurses, midwives, and health visitors will face. Whether you're raising concerns about a child's welfare, discussing domestic abuse with a vulnerable adult, or escalating a risk to a multidisciplinary team, these moments require careful communication, legal awareness, and emotional intelligence.

Understanding Safeguarding Duties

Under the **Care Act 2014** and **Children Act 1989/2004**, all healthcare professionals have a duty to:

- Recognise signs of abuse, neglect, or exploitation.
- Respond appropriately and proportionately.
- Refer concerns to safeguarding teams or local authorities.

Safeguarding applies to both children and adults at risk, including those with disabilities, mental health needs, or cognitive impairments. Nurses must be alert to physical, emotional, sexual, financial, and institutional abuse—and understand how to act when concerns arise.

How to Communicate Risk Effectively

Communicating risk is not about creating fear—it's about enabling informed decisions and protecting safety. Key principles include:

- **Clarity**: Use plain, non-technical language. Avoid jargon or euphemisms.
- **Sensitivity**: Acknowledge emotions and avoid blame. Focus

on safety and support.

- **Transparency**: Be honest about what will happen next, including referrals or documentation.
- **Documentation**: Record concerns factually, avoiding assumptions or subjective language.

Example:

"I'm concerned about what you've shared today, and I want to make sure you're safe. I may need to speak with our safeguarding team so we can explore the best way to support you."

Navigating Difficult Dynamics

Safeguarding conversations often involve complex relationships and power dynamics. Families may feel judged, defensive, or fearful. Patients may be reluctant to disclose abuse or may lack capacity to protect themselves. Nurses must:

- Use structured tools like **SBAR** (Situation, Background, Assessment, Recommendation) to communicate concerns clearly.
- Involve safeguarding leads, social workers, or multidisciplinary teams early.
- Be prepared for emotional reactions—anger, denial, distress—and respond with empathy and professionalism.

Safeguarding and Capacity

When a person lacks capacity, safeguarding decisions must be made in their **best interests**, following the **Mental Capacity Act (2005)**. This includes:

- Considering the least restrictive option.

- Involving advocates or family members where appropriate.
- Documenting the rationale for decisions clearly.

Supporting Yourself

Safeguarding conversations can be emotionally taxing. Nurses should:

- Debrief with colleagues or supervisors.
- Use reflective practice to process emotional impact.
- Seek support from safeguarding leads or psychological services when needed.

For practical guidance, see Appendix 4: Safeguarding Conversation Checklist and Appendix 5: SBAR Template for Safeguarding Concerns.

Working with Young People and Vulnerable Adults

Conversations with young people and vulnerable adults require a heightened level of sensitivity, legal awareness, and emotional intelligence. These individuals may face barriers to understanding, expressing themselves, or asserting their rights—making the nurse's role as communicator, advocate, and protector especially vital.

Who Is Considered Vulnerable?

A vulnerable adult is someone aged 18 or over who may be unable to protect themselves from harm or exploitation due to:

- Physical or mental illness
- Learning disabilities
- Age-related frailty
- Substance misuse
- Social isolation or dependency

Young people aged 16–18 occupy a unique legal and developmental space. While they may have rights to consent and autonomy, they may also be subject to safeguarding procedures and capacity assessments under the **Mental Capacity Act (2005)** and **Children Act (1989/2004)**.

Assessing Capacity in Young People

Young people aged 16 and over are presumed to have capacity unless proven otherwise. However, nurses must consider:

- Cognitive development and emotional maturity

- Influence of peers, family, or coercive relationships
- Ability to understand and weigh risks

When capacity is in doubt, a structured assessment should be carried out, and decisions made in the young person's best interests. Involving parents or guardians may be appropriate—but only with the young person's consent or when legally required.

Communicating Effectively

Young people and vulnerable adults may struggle with abstract concepts, medical jargon, or emotionally charged topics. Nurses should:

- Use age-appropriate language and visual aids
- Allow extra time for questions and processing
- Check understanding using teach-back methods
- Create a safe, non-judgmental space for disclosure

In community settings, health visitors may notice subtle signs of distress, neglect, or coercion. Building trust over time is essential, especially when working with families or in safeguarding contexts.

Safeguarding Considerations

When working with young people or vulnerable adults, safeguarding concerns may arise around:

- Domestic abuse
- Sexual exploitation
- Self-harm or suicidal ideation
- Neglect or financial abuse

Nurses must be prepared to:

- Recognise signs of harm or manipulation
- Escalate concerns through appropriate safeguarding channels
- Document disclosures factually and sensitively
- Involve multidisciplinary teams and advocacy services

Building Trust and Advocacy

Trust is the foundation of effective communication. Nurses should:

- Respect autonomy and confidentiality (within legal limits)
- Advocate for the individual's voice in care planning
- Challenge discriminatory or dismissive attitudes in teams
- Use supervision to reflect on emotional impact and ethical dilemmas

Safeguarding Scenario: "He's Just Quiet"

Scenario

During a routine school health visit, Nurse L meets with 15-year-old Jamie, who has been referred due to frequent absences and unexplained stomach pains. Jamie is polite but withdrawn, avoids eye contact, and gives short answers. When asked about home life, he shrugs and says, "It's fine." Nurse L notices bruising on his forearm, which Jamie attributes to "messing around with mates."

The school staff describe Jamie as "just quiet" and say he's always been a bit reserved. However, Nurse L feels uneasy. Something doesn't add up. She wonders whether to escalate the concern or wait for more evidence.

Reflection

This scenario highlights the importance of trusting professional intuition and recognising subtle signs of distress. It raises key questions:

- How do we balance respect for autonomy with the duty to protect?
- What constitutes "enough" evidence to raise a safeguarding concern?
- How do we navigate confidentiality and disclosure with young people?

Learning Points

- Vulnerability is not always visible—withdrawal, vague responses, and physical signs may indicate risk.
- Nurses must document concerns factually and escalate appropriately, even when disclosures are limited.
- Safeguarding is a process, not a one-off event. Building trust may take time.
- Supervision and peer support are essential when navigating uncertainty and emotional impact.

Conclusion

Conversations about consent, capacity, and risk are central to safe, ethical, and person-centred care. Whether you're assessing a young person's decision-making ability, discussing safeguarding concerns, or navigating complex family dynamics, these moments require clarity, compassion, and confidence.

By understanding the legal frameworks—such as the Mental Capacity Act—and applying structured communication strategies, nurses, midwives, and health visitors can uphold autonomy while protecting safety. These conversations are not just clinical—they are relational, ethical, and deeply human.

When professionals speak clearly and listen deeply, they empower individuals, protect vulnerable people, and strengthen trust in the care system.

Part II: Conversations with Colleagues and Managers

Chapter 4: Addressing Gossip, Harassment, and Bullying.

Workplace culture has a direct impact on wellbeing, safety, and professional integrity. In healthcare settings, gossip, harassment, and bullying can erode trust, damage team cohesion, and compromise patient care. Yet these behaviours often go unchallenged, hidden behind humour, hierarchy, or fear of retaliation.

This chapter explores how nurses, midwives, and health visitors can address harmful behaviours with confidence and compassion. It introduces assertiveness techniques, strategies for speaking up safely, and the role of HR and professional bodies in creating a culture of dignity and respect. Because challenging misconduct isn't just interpersonal—it's a professional imperative.

Assertiveness Techniques

"Assertiveness is not about being loud—it's about being clear, calm, and courageous."

In nursing and healthcare environments, assertiveness is a vital skill for addressing inappropriate behaviour such as gossip, harassment, or bullying. It allows professionals to speak up respectfully, maintain boundaries, and protect psychological safety—without escalating conflict or compromising professionalism.

Assertiveness is especially important when confronting behaviours that undermine team cohesion or violate dignity. It empowers nurses, midwives, and health visitors to challenge misconduct while preserving relationships and emotional wellbeing.

What Assertiveness Is—and Isn't

- **Assertiveness is**: clear, respectful, confident communication that protects your rights and values.
- **Assertiveness is not**: aggression, passivity, or manipulation.

Assertive communication helps you:

- Express concerns without blame.
- Set boundaries without hostility.
- Challenge behaviour without personal attacks.

Core Assertiveness Strategies

1. "I" Statements

Use "I" statements to express how behaviour affects you, without sounding accusatory.

- *"I feel uncomfortable when conversations turn personal in a negative way."*
- *"I'd prefer not to be part of that discussion—it feels inappropriate."*

This technique reduces defensiveness and keeps the focus on impact rather than intent.

2. Broken Record Technique

Repeat your point calmly and consistently if met with resistance or deflection.

- *"I understand, but I still feel this needs to be addressed."*
- *"I hear what you're saying, but I'm not comfortable with that behaviour."*

This is especially useful when dealing with persistent gossip or dismissive responses.

3. Fogging

Acknowledge criticism without agreeing or escalating.

- *"That's your view—I see it differently."*
- *"You may not agree, but I still feel it's important to speak up."*

Fogging helps you stay grounded and avoid being drawn into emotional conflict.

4. Boundary Setting

Clearly define what is acceptable and what is not.

- *"I'm here to work collaboratively. I'd appreciate it if we could keep things professional."*
- *"I'm not comfortable with that comment. Let's focus on the task."*

Boundaries protect your emotional safety and reinforce respectful workplace norms.

Assertiveness in Action: Healthcare Scenarios

Scenario: Gossip in the Break Room

A colleague repeatedly makes sarcastic remarks about another team member's appearance or accent.

Assertive Response:

"I don't think those comments are fair or helpful. Let's keep our conversations respectful."

Scenario: Undermining Behaviour

A senior colleague dismisses your input during handover.

Assertive Response:

"I'd like to finish sharing my observations—they're relevant to the patient's care."

Scenario: Inappropriate 'Banter'

A colleague jokes about a junior staff member's cultural background.

Assertive Response:

"That kind of humour can be hurtful. I think we need to be more mindful of how we speak."

Emotional Intelligence and Assertiveness

Assertiveness is not just about words—it's about emotional regulation and presence. Key emotional skills include:

- **Staying calm**: Manage your own emotional reactions to stay composed.
- **Listening actively**: Show empathy while maintaining boundaries.
- **Responding, not reacting**: Pause before speaking to ensure clarity and professionalism.
- **Being aware of neurodiversity and cultural differences**: Tailor your approach to individual needs and avoid assumptions.

Assertiveness Checklist

Before speaking up:

- Know the facts—document incidents clearly.
- Choose a private, safe space for the conversation.
- Prepare emotionally—use breathing or grounding techniques.
- Check relevant policies (e.g. dignity at work, whistleblowing).

During the conversation:

- Use "I" statements and stay calm.
- Focus on behaviour, not personality.
- Listen actively and avoid interrupting.

- Take breaks if emotions escalate.

After the conversation:

- Document outcomes and agreed actions.
- Seek supervision or HR support if needed.
- Reflect on what went well and what could improve.

Speaking Up Safely

"Courage doesn't mean you're not afraid—it means you speak up anyway, with care and clarity."

In healthcare settings, speaking up about inappropriate behaviour—whether it's gossip, harassment, or bullying—is essential for maintaining a safe, respectful, and inclusive environment. Yet many professionals hesitate, fearing retaliation, emotional fallout, or being misunderstood. Creating psychological safety and using structured approaches can help nurses, midwives, and health visitors raise concerns confidently and professionally.

Why Speaking Up Matters

Avoiding difficult conversations can:

- Reinforce toxic behaviours
- Undermine team morale
- Compromise patient safety
- Erode professional integrity

Speaking up is not about confrontation—it's about accountability, dignity, and care.

Barriers to Speaking Up

From both toolkits, common barriers include:

- Fear of emotional reactions or escalation
- Anxiety about damaging relationships
- Lack of confidence or communication skills

- Uncertainty about policies or procedures
- Cultural or neurodiversity-related misunderstandings

Recognising these barriers helps professionals prepare and seek support before initiating a conversation.

Strategies for Speaking Up Safely

1. Prepare Thoughtfully

- **Know the facts**: Document incidents clearly and objectively.
- **Check policies**: Review dignity at work, whistleblowing, and safeguarding procedures.
- **Choose the right time and place**: Private, calm settings reduce defensiveness.
- **Plan your message**: Use a script or notes to stay focused.

2. Use Structured Communication Tools

- **SBAR (Situation, Background, Assessment, Recommendation)**: Ideal for framing concerns in clinical language *(Appendix 3)*
- **NURSE or VALUE frameworks**: Useful for emotionally sensitive conversations.
- **Open and closed questions**: Start with open questions to explore, then use closed questions to clarify.

3. Stay Emotionally Grounded

- **Regulate your emotions**: Use breathing techniques or grounding strategies.
- **Remain calm**: Avoid raising your voice or reacting defensively.

- **Pause if needed**: If emotions escalate, suggest a break or follow-up meeting.

4. Focus on Behaviour, Not Personality

- *"I've noticed some comments that feel inappropriate."*
- *"I'm concerned about how this might affect team dynamics."*

Avoid labels like "bully" or "toxic"—focus on specific actions and their impact.

Example Conversation Starters

- *"I wanted to raise something that's been bothering me—can we talk privately?"*
- *"I've noticed some behaviours that feel exclusionary. I think it's important we address it."*
- *"I'm not comfortable with that comment. Can we keep things respectful?"*

These openers signal concern without blame, creating space for dialogue.

When to Escalate

If direct conversation doesn't resolve the issue—or if the behaviour is serious—escalation may be necessary.

Options include:

- Speaking with a line manager or supervisor
- Contacting HR or Employee Relations
- Using whistleblowing or safeguarding channels
- Seeking support from professional bodies (e.g. NMC)

Always document concerns factually and seek guidance if unsure.

Support Systems

- **Equality and Diversity Teams**: Advice on neurodiversity and discrimination
- **Reflective Supervision**: Emotional processing and professional growth
- **Staff Psychological Support Services**
- **Employee Assistance Programmes**

Speaking up is emotionally demanding; support is essential for resilience and wellbeing.

Role of HR and Professional Bodies

"Support systems exist not to punish—but to protect, guide, and uphold professional standards."

When gossip, harassment, or bullying occurs in healthcare settings, it's essential to know where to turn. Speaking up is the first step—but knowing how to escalate concerns and access support is equally important. Human Resources (HR) departments and professional bodies like the **Nursing and Midwifery Council (NMC)** play a vital role in ensuring that concerns are addressed fairly, confidentially, and in line with professional standards.

The Role of Human Resources (HR)

HR teams are responsible for:

- **Investigating complaints**: Ensuring fair, confidential, and timely resolution.
- **Enforcing policies**: Including dignity at work, whistleblowing, and grievance procedures.
- **Supporting mediation**: Facilitating conversations between staff to resolve conflict.
- **Protecting wellbeing**: Referring staff to psychological support or occupational health services.

When to involve HR:

- If informal resolution fails
- If the behaviour is repeated or escalates
- If the issue involves discrimination, harassment, or

safeguarding concerns

How to approach HR:

- Document incidents clearly and factually
- Request a confidential meeting
- Refer to relevant policies (e.g. bullying and harassment, equality and diversity)

The Role of Professional Bodies

The **Nursing and Midwifery Council (NMC)** sets the standards for professional behaviour and accountability. It provides guidance, support, and regulatory oversight when serious concerns arise.

Key responsibilities of the NMC:

- Upholding the Code of Conduct
- Investigating fitness to practise concerns
- Providing ethical guidance and professional standards
- Supporting whistleblowers and safeguarding professionals

When to contact the NMC:

- If misconduct compromises patient safety or professional integrity
- If internal resolution fails and the issue is serious
- If you need guidance on ethical dilemmas or professional boundaries

- **Other bodies to consider:**

- **Trade unions**: Offer representation and advice during grievance processes

- **Safeguarding boards**: For concerns involving vulnerable individuals
- **Occupational health**: For emotional or psychological support

Creating a Culture of Accountability

HR and professional bodies are not just reactive—they help shape a culture where dignity, respect, and safety are prioritised.

Managers and leaders should:

- Model respectful behaviour
- Encourage open dialogue
- Provide training on communication and conflict resolution
- Support staff through supervision and reflective practice

Staff should feel empowered to:

- Raise concerns early
- Seek support without fear
- Trust that their voice matters

Navigating Support Systems

Conversation Starters:

- *"I'd like to speak with HR about a concern I've been experiencing."*
- *"Can we review the dignity at work policy together?"*
- *"I'm unsure how to escalate this—can you guide me?"*

Support Resources:

- HR and Employee Relations teams
- NMC Code and guidance
- Occupational health and counselling services
- Trade unions and safeguarding leads
- Equality and Diversity teams

Conclusion

Gossip, harassment, and bullying are not just interpersonal issues—they are professional risks that undermine safety, wellbeing, and team cohesion. Nurses, midwives, and health visitors must feel empowered to challenge these behaviours with clarity, assertiveness, and support.

By using structured communication techniques, understanding the role of HR and professional bodies, and fostering a culture of psychological safety, healthcare professionals can help create respectful, inclusive environments where everyone feels valued. Speaking up is not a disruption—it's a commitment to care, integrity, and professional standards.

Chapter 5: Managing Workload and Burnout

"*You can't pour from an empty cup. Caring for others starts with caring for yourself.*"

Healthcare professionals are known for their resilience—but even the most dedicated nurses, midwives, and health visitors can reach a breaking point. The emotional intensity of care, combined with high workloads, lone working, and systemic pressures, can lead to burnout, moral distress, and reduced job satisfaction.

This chapter explores how to recognise and respond to burnout, manage workload effectively, and create a culture of support through supervision, peer connection, and compassionate leadership. It also offers practical strategies for raising concerns constructively and sustaining wellbeing in demanding environments. Because caring for others starts with caring for ourselves.

Understanding Burnout in Healthcare

Burnout is more than feeling tired—it's a state of emotional, physical, and professional exhaustion caused by prolonged stress, high demands, and insufficient support. In nursing, burnout can manifest as:

- Emotional detachment from patients
- Reduced empathy or compassion fatigue
- Cynicism or irritability
- Decreased job satisfaction
- Physical symptoms like headaches, insomnia, or fatigue

Burnout doesn't just affect the individual—it impacts team dynamics, patient safety, and retention across the healthcare system.

Contributing Factors

Common contributors to burnout include:

- **High workload and staffing shortages**
- **Emotional intensity of care** (especially in palliative, safeguarding, or trauma settings)
- **Lack of control or autonomy**
- **Poor team communication or unresolved conflict**
- **Inadequate supervision or support**
- **Moral distress**—feeling unable to act according to professional values

Health visitors and community nurses may face additional challenges, including lone working, safeguarding pressures, and blurred boundaries between personal and professional life.

Recognising the Signs

Burnout often develops gradually. Key indicators include:

- Feeling overwhelmed or constantly behind
- Loss of motivation or joy in work
- Withdrawing from colleagues or patients
- Increased errors or forgetfulness
- Feeling "numb" or emotionally exhausted

Early recognition is essential. Reflective practice, supervision, and peer support can help identify and address burnout before it escalates.

Strategies for Managing Workload

1. Prioritisation and Boundaries

- Use tools like the **Eisenhower Matrix** to distinguish urgent vs. important tasks.
- Set realistic goals for each shift or visit.
- Learn to say "no" or delegate when appropriate.

2. Time Management

- Block time for documentation, breaks, and supervision.
- Use checklists or digital tools to streamline tasks.
- Avoid multitasking during emotionally intense conversations.

3. Team Communication

- Share workload concerns in team meetings or handovers.

- Use SBAR to escalate safely and clearly.
- Support colleagues by checking in and offering help when possible.

Preventing and Recovering from Burnout

1. Supervision and Reflective Practice

- Schedule regular supervision—clinical, managerial, or reflective.
- Use models like **Gibbs** or **Schön** to process emotional experiences.
- Reflect on what energises vs. drains you in your role.

2. Emotional Self-Care

- Practice grounding techniques (e.g., breathing, mindfulness).
- Take breaks—even short ones—to reset.
- Use journaling or creative outlets to process stress.

3. Organisational Support

- Access occupational health or psychological support services.
- Use health passports or wellbeing plans to communicate needs.
- Advocate for safe staffing, fair rotas, and protected time for supervision.

CASE STUDY: "I'M JUST So Tired"

Scenario: Nurse B, working in a busy community safeguarding role, begins to feel emotionally drained. She notices she's avoiding calls, forgetting details, and feeling resentful toward families. In supervision, she breaks down and says, "I'm just so tired. I don't know if I can keep doing this."

Response:

- Her supervisor validates her feelings and explores workload adjustments.
- Together, they identify tasks that can be delegated and schedule protected time for reflection.
- Nurse B is referred to occupational health and begins attending peer support sessions.

Outcome:

- With support, Nurse B regains clarity and confidence. She adjusts her caseload, re-engages with supervision, and begins to feel more grounded in her role.

For practical guidance see Appendix 6: Managing Workload and Burnout Toolkit

Leading Through Burnout: Supporting Your Team

"*Leadership is not about being in charge—it's about caring for those in your charge.*"

In healthcare, team leaders—whether ward managers, senior nurses, or safeguarding leads—play a critical role in preventing and responding to burnout. Leadership is not just about managing tasks—it's about fostering emotional safety, modelling resilience, and creating a culture where wellbeing is prioritised.

Recognising Burnout in Others

Team leaders should be alert to signs of burnout in colleagues, including:

- Withdrawal or irritability
- Increased errors or forgetfulness
- Emotional outbursts or detachment
- Avoidance of patients or responsibilities
- Frequent sickness absence or lateness

These signs may be subtle. Regular check-ins, supervision, and informal conversations can help surface concerns early.

Creating a Supportive Team Culture

1. Normalise Conversations About Wellbeing

- Start meetings with a "how are you really?" check-in.
- Share your own challenges to model vulnerability and

openness.
- Encourage reflective practice and emotional debriefing.

2. Protect Time for Supervision and Breaks

- Schedule regular supervision for all staff—not just those in crisis.
- Ensure breaks are taken and respected.
- Advocate for protected time for documentation, reflection, and recovery.

3. Respond to Concerns with Compassion and Action

- Listen actively and without judgement.
- Validate emotional experiences: *"That sounds incredibly tough—thank you for sharing."*
- Explore practical adjustments: caseload changes, flexible working, peer support.

Leadership Behaviours That Prevent Burnout

- **Clarity**: Set clear expectations and boundaries.
- **Empathy**: Understand the emotional demands of frontline work.
- **Consistency**: Follow through on support and supervision commitments.
- **Advocacy**: Speak up for staffing, resources, and wellbeing initiatives.
- **Reflection**: Use feedback and supervision to improve your own leadership style.

Case Study: "We're All Running on Empty"

Scenario: A safeguarding team reports rising stress levels and emotional fatigue. The team leader notices increased sickness absence and tension in meetings.

Response:

- The leader arranges a reflective supervision session for the whole team.
- They review caseloads, redistribute tasks, and introduce weekly wellbeing check-ins.
- The leader also advocates for additional staffing and liaises with occupational health.

Outcome:

- Staff feel heard and supported. Absence rates drop, and team morale improves.
- The leader reflects on their own role and commits to ongoing emotional leadership.

For practical guidance see Appendix 7: Leading Through Burnout Toolkit

RAISING CONCERNS CONSTRUCTIVELY

"Speaking up is not about blame—it's about building safer, stronger systems."

In healthcare, raising concerns about workload, safety, or wellbeing is a professional responsibility. Yet many nurses, midwives, and health visitors hesitate—fearing conflict, dismissal, or being labelled as "difficult." Constructive communication helps transform concerns into opportunities for improvement, collaboration, and care.

Why Concerns Must Be Raised

Unspoken concerns can lead to:

- Unsafe staffing levels
- Missed safeguarding opportunities
- Emotional exhaustion and burnout
- Compromised patient care
- Moral injury and professional regret

The **NMC Code** emphasises the duty to speak up when care is compromised. Constructive communication ensures that concerns are heard, understood, and acted upon.

Barriers to Raising Concerns

Common barriers include:

- Fear of retaliation or being misunderstood
- Lack of confidence or communication skills
- Hierarchical dynamics or cultural norms
- Emotional fatigue or resignation
- Unclear policies or escalation routes

Recognising these barriers helps professionals prepare and seek support before speaking up.

How to Raise Concerns Constructively

1. Prepare Thoughtfully

- **Clarify the issue**: What is the concern? What impact is it having?
- **Gather evidence**: Document incidents, patterns, or risks factually.

- **Know your policies**: Review whistleblowing, safeguarding, and supervision procedures.

2. Use Structured Communication Tools

- **SBAR (Situation, Background, Assessment, Recommendation)**: Ideal for clinical and operational concerns.
- **Reflective models**: Use Gibbs or Schön to explore emotional and ethical dimensions.
- **Conversation starters**:
    - *"I've noticed something that's affecting care—can we talk about it?"*
    - *"I'm concerned about how this is impacting the team and patients."*

3. Choose the Right Setting

- Request a private, calm space for discussion.
- Avoid raising concerns in emotionally charged or public environments.
- Consider involving a supervisor, safeguarding lead, or union representative if needed.

4. Focus on Impact, Not Blame

- *"This situation is affecting patient safety and team wellbeing."*
- *"I'm raising this because I care about the quality of care we provide."*

Avoid personalising the issue—focus on behaviour, systems, and outcomes.

Escalating When Necessary

If concerns are not resolved informally, escalation may be required.

Options include:

- Line manager or clinical lead
- HR or Employee Relations
- Safeguarding teams
- Whistleblowing channels
- Professional bodies (e.g. NMC)

Always document concerns clearly and seek guidance if unsure.

Case Study: "I Don't Feel Safe"

Scenario: A health visitor feels overwhelmed by her caseload and is worried that safeguarding risks are being missed. She's hesitant to speak up, fearing she'll be seen as incompetent.

Response:

- She uses SBAR to frame her concern and requests a supervision session.
- Her manager listens, validates her concern, and reviews caseload distribution.
- Together, they escalate the issue to senior leadership and advocate for staffing support.

Outcome:

- The team receives temporary support and reviews safeguarding protocols.
- The health visitor feels heard and empowered to continue raising concerns.

For practical guidance see Appendix 8: Raising Concerns Constructively Toolkit

Peer Support and Supervision

"*Supervision is not a luxury—it's a lifeline. Peer support is not a bonus—it's a buffer against burnout.*"

In emotionally demanding healthcare environments, peer support and supervision are essential tools for sustaining wellbeing, professional integrity, and team cohesion. They offer space to reflect, decompress, and grow—especially when workload and emotional intensity threaten resilience.

What Is Supervision?

Supervision in nursing can take several forms:

- **Clinical supervision**: Focused on practice, decision-making, and standards.
- **Managerial supervision**: Focused on performance, accountability, and caseload.
- **Reflective supervision**: Focused on emotional processing, ethical dilemmas, and professional growth.

Reflective supervision is particularly valuable in safeguarding, palliative care, and lone-working roles, where emotional labour is high and boundaries are complex.

Benefits of Supervision

- Reduces emotional fatigue and moral distress
- Enhances decision-making and confidence
- Supports ethical reflection and safeguarding practice
- Strengthens team relationships and psychological safety

- Promotes learning, growth, and resilience

Supervision is not just for those in crisis—it's a proactive tool for sustainable practice.

What Is Peer Support?

Peer support involves informal or structured connection with colleagues to share experiences, offer empathy, and reduce isolation. It can take the form of:

- Informal chats or debriefs
- Peer mentoring or buddy systems
- Group reflective sessions
- Online forums or virtual check-ins

Health visitors and community nurses, who often work alone, benefit especially from scheduled peer contact.

Creating a Culture of Support

1. Normalise Supervision and Peer Support

- Include supervision in job plans and rotas.
- Encourage staff to request support early—not just in crisis.
- Celebrate peer support as a sign of professionalism, not weakness.

2. Make It Accessible

- Offer flexible formats: in-person, virtual, one-to-one, group.
- Protect time for supervision and peer connection.
- Use health passports or wellbeing plans to tailor support.

3. Use Structured Models

- **Gibbs Reflective Cycle**: Explore feelings, actions, and learning.
- **Schön's Reflective Practice**: Reflect-in-action and reflect-on-action.
- **SAFE or RESTORE models**: For trauma-informed supervision.

Case Study: "I Didn't Realise I Needed This"

Scenario: A newly qualified nurse joins a safeguarding team and begins to feel overwhelmed. She's unsure whether her emotional reactions are "normal" and fears being judged.

Response:

- Her supervisor introduces reflective supervision and pairs her with a peer mentor.
- In supervision, she explores her emotional responses and learns strategies for regulation.
- Her mentor shares similar experiences, helping her feel less alone.

Outcome:

- The nurse gains confidence, emotional clarity, and a sense of belonging.
- She begins to use supervision proactively and supports others in doing the same.

For practical guidance see Appendix 9: Peer Support and Supervision Toolkit

Conclusion

Burnout is not a personal failure—it's a signal that something needs to change. In nursing, midwifery, and health visiting, managing workload and emotional intensity is essential for safe, sustainable practice. This chapter has explored how to recognise burnout, raise concerns constructively, and build resilience through supervision, peer support, and compassionate leadership.

By prioritising wellbeing, setting boundaries, and fostering a culture of care, healthcare professionals can protect themselves and each other. Because when we care for the carers, we strengthen the entire system.

Chapter 6: Challenging Unsafe Practices

"Safety isn't just physical—it's psychological. Speaking up protects patients, teams, and trust."

In healthcare, unsafe practices can arise from errors, omissions, poor communication, or systemic failures. Nurses, midwives, and health visitors are often the first to notice when something isn't right—but speaking up can feel risky. Challenging unsafe practices requires courage, clarity, and a culture that supports transparency.

This chapter explores how to raise concerns constructively, use structured communication tools like SBAR, and understand the legal and ethical frameworks of whistleblowing and duty of candour. It begins with the foundation of all safe communication: **psychological safety**.

Psychological Safety in Teams

"When people feel safe to speak, teams become safer for everyone."

Psychological safety refers to a team climate where individuals feel safe to express concerns, ask questions, admit mistakes, and challenge decisions—without fear of humiliation, retaliation, or exclusion. In healthcare, psychological safety is essential for preventing harm, improving outcomes, and fostering learning.

Why It Matters

When psychological safety is low:

- Staff may stay silent about errors or risks
- Junior colleagues may fear challenging senior staff
- Mistakes may be repeated or hidden
- Emotional distress and moral injury increase

When psychological safety is high:

- Concerns are raised early and constructively
- Teams learn from mistakes and improve together
- Staff feel valued, respected, and supported
- Patient safety and care quality improve

Barriers to Psychological Safety

- **Hierarchical cultures**: Fear of challenging authority
- **Blame culture**: Focus on fault rather than learning
- **Lack of supervision**: No space to reflect or decompress
- **Discrimination or bias**: Some voices are dismissed or

marginalised
- **Emotional fatigue**: Staff feel too overwhelmed to speak up

Health visitors and community nurses may face additional challenges due to lone working, limited peer contact, and emotionally complex safeguarding cases.

Creating a Safe Team Culture

1. Model Vulnerability and Openness

- Share your own mistakes and learning moments
- Invite feedback and questions
- Respond to concerns with curiosity, not defensiveness

2. Use Inclusive Communication

- Encourage all voices in handovers and meetings
- Use open questions: *"What are we missing?"*, *"Does anyone see it differently?"*
- Avoid interrupting or dismissing junior staff

3. Protect Time for Reflection

- Schedule regular supervision and debriefs
- Use reflective models to explore emotional and ethical challenges
- Create space for emotional processing—not just clinical review

4. Respond Supportively to Concerns

- Thank staff for raising issues—even if uncomfortable
- Focus on behaviour and systems, not blame

- Follow up with action and feedback

Case Study: "I Didn't Feel I Could Say Anything"

Scenario: During a busy ward shift, a junior nurse notices a medication error but hesitates to speak up. The senior nurse is stressed and dismissive. Later, the error is discovered, and the junior nurse feels guilty and ashamed.

Reflection:

- What prevented the nurse from speaking up?
- How could the team have created more psychological safety?
- What systems could support early intervention?

Learning Points:

- Psychological safety must be intentional and consistent
- Leaders set the tone—but everyone contributes
- Speaking up should be seen as a strength, not a threat

Whistleblowing and Duty of Candour

"Transparency is not optional—it's a professional obligation."

In nursing, midwifery, and health visiting, the duty to speak up when care is compromised is not just ethical—it's legal. Whistleblowing and the duty of candour are two key frameworks that protect patients, uphold professional standards, and support staff in raising concerns about unsafe practices.

What Is Whistleblowing?

Whistleblowing refers to the act of reporting unsafe, illegal, or unethical practices within an organisation. It is protected by law under the **Public Interest Disclosure Act (1998)** and supported by professional codes such as the **NMC Code**.

Examples of whistleblowing concerns:

- Unsafe staffing levels
- Medication errors being concealed
- Abuse or neglect of patients
- Fraud or misuse of resources
- Discrimination or harassment

Whistleblowing is distinct from raising a personal grievance—it must be in the public interest and relate to safety, legality, or ethics.

What Is the Duty of Candour?

The **Duty of Candour** is a legal requirement for health professionals and organisations to be open and honest when something goes wrong with a patient's care. It applies when:

- A patient suffers harm or distress due to a mistake or omission
- The incident meets the threshold for moderate or severe harm

Key responsibilities under the Duty of Candour:

- Inform the patient or family promptly
- Apologise sincerely
- Explain what happened and what will be done
- Document the conversation and follow-up actions

The duty of candour promotes trust, learning, and accountability. It is not about blame—it's about integrity.

How to Speak Up Safely

1. Know Your Policies

- Review your organisation's whistleblowing and candour procedures
- Understand who to report to and how concerns are escalated
- Use internal reporting channels before going external (unless unsafe to do so)

2. Document Clearly

- Record incidents factually, avoiding emotional or accusatory language
- Include dates, times, witnesses, and impact
- Keep records secure and confidential

3. Use Support Systems

- Seek guidance from a supervisor, safeguarding lead, or union representative
- Access occupational health or psychological support if needed
- Use anonymous reporting channels if available

4. Protect Yourself

- Know your rights under whistleblowing legislation
- Avoid discussing concerns publicly or on social media
- Maintain professionalism and confidentiality throughout

Case Study: "I Knew I Had to Say Something"

Scenario: A midwife notices repeated medication errors on her ward, but they are being quietly corrected without documentation. She feels uneasy and worries about patient safety.

Response:

- She documents the incidents and raises the concern with her line manager.
- When no action is taken, she contacts the organisation's whistleblowing lead.
- The issue is investigated, and systems are improved. She is supported throughout.

Outcome:

- Patient safety improves, and the midwife is recognised for her professionalism.
- The team receives training on duty of candour and error reporting.

SBAR for Structured Communication

"Clarity saves lives. Structure gives confidence."

In high-pressure healthcare environments, communication errors can lead to serious consequences. Whether you're escalating a concern, reporting an incident, or handing over care, structured communication helps ensure that vital information is shared clearly, consistently, and professionally.

One of the most widely used tools for this purpose is **SBAR**—a simple, effective framework for speaking up and sharing information.

What Is SBAR?

SBAR stands for:

- **S**ituation: What is happening right now?
- **B**ackground: What is the relevant context?
- **A**ssessment: What do you think the problem is?
- **R**ecommendation: What do you suggest should happen?

Originally developed in the military and adapted for healthcare, SBAR is now used across hospitals, community teams, and safeguarding settings to support safe, assertive communication.

Why SBAR Works

- Reduces ambiguity and confusion
- Helps junior staff speak up with confidence
- Supports escalation of concerns without emotional overload
- Encourages clinical reasoning and accountability

- Promotes shared understanding across multidisciplinary teams

SBAR is especially useful when challenging unsafe practices, raising safeguarding concerns, or communicating under pressure.

Using SBAR in Practice

Example 1: Medication Error

- **S**: "I'm calling about Mrs. K in Bay 3—she was given the wrong dose of insulin."
- **B**: "She's a diabetic patient admitted this morning. Her chart shows 6 units, but 12 were administered."
- **A**: "She's now showing signs of hypoglycaemia—sweating, confusion."
- **R**: "I recommend immediate review and monitoring. Can you attend now?"

Example 2: Safeguarding Concern

- **S**: "I have a concern about a child I visited today—Jamie, age 5."
- **B**: "He lives with his mother, who appeared intoxicated during the visit. Jamie had bruises and seemed withdrawn."
- **A**: "I believe there may be a safeguarding risk—possible neglect or physical harm."
- **R**: "I recommend escalating to the safeguarding team and arranging a joint visit."

Tips for Effective SBAR Use

- Prepare before speaking, jot down key points

- Stay calm and focused, especially under stress
- Use professional language and avoid blame
- Be clear about what you need—don't leave it vague
- Follow up with documentation and supervision

Toolkit: SBAR for Challenging Unsafe Practices

Conversation Prompts:

- *"Can I use SBAR to explain a concern I have?"*
- *"I'd like to recommend a course of action based on what I've observed."*

Support Resources:

- SBAR templates and training
- Supervision for debriefing and reflection
- Safeguarding leads and escalation pathways
- NMC Code and organisational policies

Conclusion

Challenging unsafe practices is not just a professional responsibility—it's a courageous act of care. Whether you're raising concerns about a medication error, escalating a safeguarding issue, or speaking up about systemic risks, your voice matters. It protects patients, strengthens teams, and upholds the integrity of the healthcare system.

This chapter has explored the foundations of safe communication: psychological safety, structured tools like SBAR, and the legal and ethical frameworks of whistleblowing and duty of candour. These are not just policies—they are practices that shape culture, build trust, and save lives.

As a nurse, midwife, or health visitor, you are not alone. Support systems exist to help you speak up safely, reflect deeply, and lead with integrity. When you challenge unsafe practices, you don't just prevent harm—you model the kind of leadership our profession needs.

"When we speak up, we don't just protect others—we honour our values, our training, and our humanity."

Part III: Navigating Bias, Advocacy, and Power Dynamics

Chapter 7: Talking About Racism and Bias

Conversations about racism and bias are among the most sensitive and necessary in healthcare. For nurses, midwives, and health visitors, these discussions are not just about interpersonal dynamics—they are about safety, dignity, and equity in care. Whether addressing microaggressions in the workplace, advocating for inclusive practices, or challenging discriminatory behaviour, speaking up requires courage, clarity, and cultural humility.

Healthcare professionals often work in diverse teams and serve communities with varied backgrounds, beliefs, and experiences. Yet, systemic inequalities and unconscious bias can shape interactions in ways that undermine trust and perpetuate harm. Silence in the face of racism—whether overt or subtle—can erode psychological safety, damage team cohesion, and compromise patient outcomes.

This chapter offers practical frameworks for initiating and sustaining sensitive dialogue about racism and bias. It explores the impact of microaggressions, the role of allyship, and strategies for creating inclusive team cultures. You'll learn how to speak up with professionalism and empathy, how to support colleagues experiencing discrimination, and how to foster environments where every voice is valued.

Talking about racism is not a disruption to care—it is part of it. It is how we uphold the values of equity, respect, and compassion that define our profession. With the right tools and support, nurses can lead these conversations with integrity and impact.

Frameworks for Sensitive Dialogue

Talking about racism and bias in nursing is not just about identifying problems—it's about creating space for honest, respectful, and transformative dialogue. These conversations can be emotionally charged, especially when they involve lived experiences of discrimination, unconscious bias, or systemic inequality. Nurses, midwives, and health visitors need structured frameworks that support clarity, empathy, and psychological safety.

Why Frameworks Matter

Sensitive conversations often falter without structure. People may feel defensive, misunderstood, or overwhelmed. Frameworks offer a roadmap—helping professionals stay grounded, listen actively, and respond with compassion. They also support accountability, ensuring that concerns are addressed rather than dismissed.

In healthcare, where time is limited and emotions run high, having a reliable approach can make the difference between escalation and resolution.

The LEAPS Framework for Anti-Racist Dialogue

The **LEAPS** framework is designed to support conversations about racism, bias, and inclusion in professional settings:

- **L – Listen**: Create space for the person to share their experience without interruption. Use active listening techniques and avoid rushing to respond.
- **E – Empathise**: Acknowledge the emotional impact of what's been shared. Validation is key: "That sounds incredibly

difficult. Thank you for trusting me with that."

- **A – Ask**: Use open-ended questions to explore the issue further. "Can you tell me more about what happened?" or "What do you need from me right now?"
- **P – Pause**: Take a moment to reflect before responding. This helps regulate emotional reactions and prevents defensiveness.
- **S – Support**: Offer practical support, whether that's raising the issue with a manager, documenting the concern, or signposting to resources.

This framework encourages emotional presence and professional responsibility. It's especially useful when responding to disclosures of microaggressions, exclusion, or discriminatory behaviour.

The BRAVE Model for Speaking Up

When initiating a conversation about bias or racism, the **BRAVE** model can help structure your approach:

- **B – Be clear**: State your concern calmly and clearly. Avoid vague language or euphemisms.
- **R – Respect boundaries**: Honour the other person's emotional space and readiness to engage.
- **A – Ask for dialogue**: Invite conversation rather than confrontation. "Would you be open to talking about something that's been on my mind?"
- **V – Validate impact**: Focus on how the behaviour or comment affected you or others, rather than assigning intent.
- **E – Explore solutions**: Collaborate on ways to move forward—whether that's team training, policy review, or personal reflection.

This model supports assertive, respectful communication and is particularly helpful when challenging behaviour from colleagues or advocating for inclusive practices.

Creating a Safe Space for Dialogue

Sensitive conversations require psychological safety. This means:

- **Avoiding blame or shame**: Focus on impact, not intent.
- **Using inclusive language**: Avoid jargon, stereotypes, or assumptions.
- **Being open to feedback**: Recognise that learning about bias is ongoing.
- **Following up**: Ensure that concerns are not just heard but acted upon.

In community settings, health visitors may need to navigate cultural misunderstandings or family dynamics with care. In hospital teams, nurses may need to challenge hierarchical norms or advocate for marginalised colleagues. In all cases, structured dialogue helps turn discomfort into growth.

Microaggressions and Allyship

In healthcare settings, racism and bias often manifest not through overt acts, but through subtle, everyday interactions known as **microaggressions**. These are brief, commonplace comments or behaviours that—intentionally or not—communicate exclusion, stereotype, or disrespect. For nurses, midwives, and health visitors, recognising and responding to microaggressions is essential for fostering inclusive, psychologically safe environments.

Understanding Microaggressions

Microaggressions can be verbal, non-verbal, or environmental. They may seem minor in isolation, but their cumulative impact can be deeply harmful, leading to stress, burnout, and a sense of invisibility among those affected.

Examples in healthcare include:

- Asking a colleague, "Where are you really from?" despite knowing they were born locally.
- Assuming a nurse of colour is a healthcare assistant or support worker.
- Commenting that someone is "too articulate" or "surprisingly professional."
- Making jokes about accents, names, or cultural practices.

These interactions often stem from unconscious bias, but their effect is real. They undermine trust, reinforce stereotypes, and contribute to a culture of exclusion.

Responding to Microaggressions

Whether you witness a microaggression or experience one yourself, responding can be difficult. Fear of conflict, retaliation, or being misunderstood may lead to silence. Yet silence can be interpreted as acceptance.

Here are some strategies for responding:

- **Name the impact**: "That comment felt dismissive and made me uncomfortable."
- **Use 'I' statements**: "I felt excluded when that was said."
- **Ask for clarification**: "Can you explain what you meant by that?"
- **Redirect the conversation**: "Let's focus on respectful language—this isn't appropriate."

In team settings, it may be helpful to follow up privately or raise concerns through supervision or HR channels. Documentation and reflection are key, especially if the behaviour is repeated or part of a wider pattern.

The Role of Allyship

Allyship is the active, ongoing practice of supporting colleagues who face discrimination or exclusion. It's not about being a saviour—it's about standing in solidarity, amplifying marginalised voices, and challenging injustice.

Effective allyship in nursing includes:

- **Speaking up**: Challenge biased comments or behaviours, even when it's uncomfortable.
- **Listening deeply**: Create space for colleagues to share their experiences without judgment.
- **Educating yourself**: Learn about racism, privilege, and

systemic inequality—don't rely on others to teach you.
- **Advocating for change**: Support inclusive policies, training, and recruitment practices.

Allyship is especially powerful when it comes from those in positions of privilege or authority. Senior nurses, managers, and educators have a responsibility to model inclusive behaviour and create environments where everyone feels safe and valued.

Building a Culture of Allyship

Allyship is not a one-off act—it's a culture. Teams that embrace allyship:

- Encourage open dialogue about bias and inclusion.
- Celebrate diversity in all its forms.
- Provide training on unconscious bias, cultural competence, and inclusive communication.
- Hold each other accountable for respectful behaviour.

In community roles, allyship may involve advocating for families facing discrimination or supporting young people navigating identity and belonging. In hospital settings, it may mean challenging exclusionary practices or supporting colleagues who feel marginalised.

When nurses act as allies, they don't just support individuals—they strengthen the entire team and improve care for all.

For practical tips see Appendix 4: Allyship Toolkit for Nurses

Creating Inclusive Team Cultures

Inclusive team cultures don't happen by accident—they are built intentionally through leadership, dialogue, and everyday actions. In nursing, midwifery, and health visiting, where collaboration and trust are essential, fostering inclusion is not just a moral imperative—it's a clinical one. Inclusive teams are safer, more resilient, and better equipped to deliver equitable care.

What Does Inclusion Look Like?

An inclusive team culture is one where:

- Everyone feels psychologically safe to speak up.
- Diverse perspectives are welcomed and respected.
- Discrimination and bias are actively challenged.
- Policies and practices reflect equity and fairness.
- Emotional wellbeing and cultural identity are supported.

Inclusion is not just about representation—it's about belonging. It means that all team members, regardless of background, feel valued, heard, and empowered to contribute.

Barriers to Inclusion in Healthcare Teams

Despite best intentions, many healthcare teams struggle with:

- **Hierarchical dynamics** that silence junior staff or marginalised voices.
- **Unconscious bias** in recruitment, supervision, or decision-making.
- **Lack of training** on cultural competence and anti-racism.

- **Fear of conflict** when addressing discriminatory behaviour.
- **Tokenism**, where diversity is celebrated superficially but not embedded in practice.

These barriers can lead to exclusion, burnout, and compromised patient care. Addressing them requires courage, reflection, and systemic change.

Strategies for Building Inclusive Cultures

Creating inclusive teams involves both individual and organisational action. Key strategies include:

1. Leadership Commitment

- Leaders must model inclusive behaviour and set clear expectations.
- Inclusion should be embedded in team values, supervision, and performance reviews.

2. Inclusive Communication

- Use language that respects identity and avoids stereotypes.
- Encourage open dialogue and feedback, especially around difficult topics.

3. Diverse Representation

- Ensure diversity in recruitment, leadership, and decision-making roles.
- Avoid tokenism by valuing lived experience and cultural insight.

4. Training and Education

- Provide regular training on unconscious bias, cultural humility, and inclusive practice.
- Use real-world scenarios and reflective exercises to deepen understanding.

5. Psychological Safety

- Create environments where staff feel safe to raise concerns without fear of retaliation.
- Use supervision and peer support to process emotional impact and build resilience.

6. Accountability and Action

- Respond promptly to reports of discrimination or exclusion.
- Review policies and practices regularly to ensure they promote equity.

The Role of Nurses in Culture Change

Nurses are uniquely positioned to influence team culture. Whether through everyday interactions, supervision, or advocacy, they can:

- Challenge exclusionary behaviour with professionalism and empathy.
- Support colleagues experiencing discrimination.
- Promote inclusive language and practices.
- Reflect on their own biases and commit to growth.

In community settings, health visitors may lead inclusion efforts by engaging with diverse families and advocating for culturally responsive care. In hospital teams, nurses can foster belonging through mentorship, peer support, and inclusive leadership.

Reflection and Sustained Practice

Inclusion is not a checklist—it's a continuous practice. Teams must reflect regularly on:

- Whose voices are heard—and whose are missing?
- How are decisions made—and who is involved?
- What assumptions shape our interactions—and how can we challenge them?

Inclusive cultures grow through reflection, dialogue, and action. When nurses lead this work, they don't just improve team dynamics—they transform care.

Case Study: "I Didn't Feel Safe Speaking Up"

Scenario

Amira is a newly qualified nurse working in a busy hospital ward. She is the only staff member from a minoritised ethnic background on her team. During handover, a senior nurse makes a dismissive comment about a patient's cultural practices, joking that "weird rituals don't belong in hospitals." The team laughs awkwardly, and the conversation moves on.

Amira feels uncomfortable but doesn't speak up. Later, she shares her concerns with a colleague, who advises her to "let it go" and "not make trouble." Over the next few weeks, Amira notices similar comments and microaggressions. She begins to withdraw, avoids team discussions, and feels increasingly isolated.

Eventually, Amira raises the issue during supervision. Her manager listens, validates her experience, and initiates a team-wide training on inclusive communication and cultural competence. The senior nurse is invited to reflect on their behaviour and receives coaching. Amira is supported through mentoring and peer check-ins.

Reflection Questions

- What barriers prevented Amira from speaking up initially?
- How did the team culture contribute to her sense of exclusion?
- What actions helped restore psychological safety and inclusion?
- How can teams proactively prevent similar situations?
- What role can supervision and leadership play in culture change?

Conclusion

Racism and bias are not just social issues—they are clinical, ethical, and organisational concerns that directly affect the quality of care, team wellbeing, and patient outcomes. For nurses, midwives, and health visitors, the responsibility to challenge discrimination and foster inclusion is part of professional integrity.

This chapter has explored how to navigate sensitive conversations about racism and bias using structured frameworks, respond to microaggressions with empathy and assertiveness, and build inclusive team cultures that support psychological safety and belonging. These are not easy tasks—but they are essential.

Speaking up is not about confrontation—it's about care. It's about creating environments where every patient is treated with dignity, every colleague feels valued, and every voice has space to be heard. Inclusion is not a destination—it's a practice. And nurses are uniquely positioned to lead it.

Whether you are initiating a difficult dialogue, supporting a colleague, or reflecting on your own biases, remember: your voice matters. When nurses speak up for equity, they don't just change conversations—they change culture.

Chapter 8: Advocating for Patients and Yourself

Advocacy is at the heart of nursing, midwifery, and health visiting. Whether you're speaking up for a patient's rights, challenging unsafe practices, or asserting your own professional boundaries, advocacy is how healthcare professionals uphold dignity, safety, and ethical care. Yet, advocating within complex systems—especially when power dynamics are at play—can feel daunting.

In multidisciplinary teams, nurses often navigate hierarchies, conflicting priorities, and emotionally charged decisions. Junior staff may hesitate to challenge senior colleagues. Community practitioners may feel isolated when raising safeguarding concerns. And many professionals struggle to advocate for themselves—especially when facing burnout, discrimination, or moral distress.

This chapter explores how to recognise and respond to power dynamics in healthcare, speak up effectively in team settings, and build the confidence and resilience needed to advocate with clarity and compassion. You'll learn practical strategies for asserting your voice, protecting patient rights, and sustaining your own wellbeing in the process.

Because advocacy isn't just about confrontation—it's about care. It's how nurses protect what matters most: safety, equity, and integrity.

Power Dynamics in Healthcare

Healthcare is a system built on collaboration—but it is also shaped by hierarchy. From hospital wards to community teams, power dynamics influence who speaks, who is heard, and how decisions are made. For nurses, midwives, and health visitors, understanding these dynamics is essential for effective advocacy.

Recognising Power Structures

Power in healthcare can be formal (based on role, seniority, or clinical authority) or informal (based on confidence, relationships, or cultural norms). It shows up in:

- Multidisciplinary meetings where doctors dominate decision-making.
- Ward environments where junior staff hesitate to challenge unsafe practices.
- Community settings where lone practitioners feel unsupported when raising concerns.

These dynamics can silence important voices—especially those of nurses working closest to patients and families.

Impact on Advocacy and Safety

When power is unbalanced, advocacy suffers. Staff may avoid speaking up due to fear of retaliation, being dismissed, or damaging relationships. This can lead to:

- Missed safeguarding opportunities.
- Unchallenged clinical errors.

- Emotional distress and moral injury.

Patients are also affected. When nurses feel unable to advocate, patient needs may be overlooked, especially in cases involving vulnerability, cultural misunderstanding, or complex care decisions.

Navigating Power with Professionalism

Advocating within power structures requires skill and strategy. Key approaches include:

- **Clarity and confidence**: Use structured communication tools (e.g., SBAR) to present concerns clearly and professionally.
- **Documentation**: Record concerns factually to support escalation and accountability.
- **Support systems**: Use supervision, peer networks, and safeguarding leads to navigate difficult dynamics.
- **Emotional regulation**: Stay grounded and composed, especially when facing resistance or dismissal.

Power dynamics are not inherently negative—but they must be recognised and managed. Nurses who understand these structures can advocate more effectively, protect patients, and support a culture of safety and respect.

Examples of Power Dynamics in Healthcare

1. Hierarchical Decision-Making

- In a multidisciplinary team meeting, a junior nurse raises concerns about a patient's discharge plan. The consultant dismisses the input without discussion, reinforcing a hierarchy where medical voices dominate and nursing perspectives are undervalued.

2. Role-Based Authority

- A health visitor identifies safeguarding concerns during a home visit but struggles to escalate them because social services question her authority compared to a GP's assessment. Her professional judgment is sidelined due to perceived status differences.

3. Cultural and Language Bias

- A nurse from a minoritised background is repeatedly asked to explain her accent or cultural practices by colleagues. Despite her clinical competence, she is treated as "other," which undermines her confidence and sense of belonging in the team.

4. Gendered Expectations

- Female nurses are expected to be nurturing and accommodating, while assertiveness is interpreted as aggression. Male colleagues are more readily accepted in leadership roles, even with similar experience levels.

5. Lone Working and Isolation

- Community nurses or health visitors working alone may feel unsupported when raising concerns, especially if their observations conflict with those of more senior or centrally located staff. This can lead to self-doubt and reluctance to advocate.

6. Informal Influence

- A senior nurse with strong relationships across the team uses informal influence to shape decisions, even when others disagree. Junior staff feel unable to challenge her due to fear of exclusion or retaliation.

Speaking Up in Multidisciplinary Teams

Multidisciplinary teams (MDTs) are the backbone of modern healthcare. They bring together professionals from different disciplines—nurses, doctors, social workers, therapists, and others—to collaborate on patient care. While this diversity of expertise is a strength, it can also create challenges when it comes to communication, hierarchy, and advocacy.

The Challenge of Speaking Up

In MDTs, nurses and health visitors may feel hesitant to voice concerns, especially when:

- Their perspective differs from that of a senior clinician.
- They fear being perceived as disruptive or inexperienced.
- Previous attempts to speak up were dismissed or ignored.

This silence can have serious consequences. When nurses don't feel safe to contribute, vital information may be missed, safeguarding concerns may go unaddressed, and patient care may suffer.

Creating Space for Nursing Voices

Nurses bring unique insights to MDTs—often based on close, sustained contact with patients and families. Their observations about emotional wellbeing, cultural dynamics, and safeguarding risks are essential to holistic care.

To speak up effectively, nurses can:

- **Use structured communication tools** like SBAR (Situation,

Background, Assessment, Recommendation) to present concerns clearly and professionally.
- **Prepare in advance** by documenting observations and identifying key points.
- **Seek allies** within the team who can support or reinforce their perspective.
- **Follow up** after meetings to ensure concerns are acknowledged and acted upon.

Navigating Resistance and Dismissal

Sometimes, speaking up is met with resistance. A nurse may be told, "That's not your role," or "We've already decided." In these moments, it's important to:

- Stay calm and grounded—emotional regulation helps maintain credibility.
- Reiterate the concern with clarity and focus on patient safety.
- Escalate appropriately—through supervision, safeguarding leads, or formal reporting channels.
- Reflect on the experience in supervision or peer support to process emotional impact.

Building a Culture of Collaboration

Effective MDTs value every voice. They create space for disagreement, encourage curiosity, and prioritise patient-centred care. Nurses can help build this culture by:

- Modelling respectful, assertive communication.
- Encouraging quieter colleagues to contribute.
- Challenging exclusionary behaviour with professionalism.
- Celebrating diverse perspectives and shared learning.

Speaking up in MDTs is not just about being heard—it's about making care safer, more inclusive, and more responsive. When nurses advocate with confidence and clarity, they elevate the entire team.

Building Confidence and Resilience

Advocacy in healthcare requires more than knowledge—it demands emotional strength, self-belief, and the ability to recover from setbacks. Whether you're challenging unsafe practices, navigating team dynamics, or asserting your own needs, confidence and resilience are essential tools for sustainable practice.

Why Confidence Matters

Confidence allows nurses, midwives, and health visitors to:

- Speak up clearly and assertively.
- Trust their clinical judgment and ethical instincts.
- Navigate complex conversations without fear of dismissal.
- Advocate for patients and themselves with professionalism.

Confidence is not arrogance—it's grounded self-assurance. It grows through experience, reflection, and support.

Common Barriers to Confidence

Many healthcare professionals struggle with:

- **Imposter syndrome**: Feeling inadequate despite competence.
- **Fear of conflict**: Avoiding advocacy to preserve harmony.
- **Past dismissal**: Being ignored or undermined in previous attempts to speak up.
- **Cultural or gender norms**: Internalised beliefs that discourage assertiveness.

These barriers can erode self-esteem and lead to silence—even when action is needed.

Strategies for Building Confidence

Confidence can be cultivated through:

1. Preparation

- Use structured frameworks (e.g., SBAR) to organise thoughts.
- Document concerns clearly to support advocacy.

2. Practice

- Role-play difficult conversations in supervision or peer groups.
- Reflect on past successes to reinforce self-belief.

3. Support

- Seek mentorship, supervision, or peer networks.
- Surround yourself with colleagues who validate and encourage your voice.

4. Self-Compassion

- Acknowledge mistakes without self-criticism.
- Recognise that growth comes through discomfort and learning.

Resilience in Advocacy

Resilience is the ability to recover, adapt, and continue advocating—even when faced with resistance, emotional strain, or systemic barriers. It involves:

- **Emotional regulation**: Staying calm and grounded under pressure.
- **Reflective practice**: Processing experiences to learn and grow.
- **Boundaries**: Protecting your wellbeing while remaining engaged.
- **Meaning making**: Connecting advocacy to personal and professional values.

Resilience doesn't mean being unaffected—it means being able to continue caring, speaking up, and leading with integrity.

Sustaining Yourself in Advocacy Work

Advocacy can be emotionally taxing. To sustain yourself:

- Schedule regular supervision or reflective sessions.
- Use journaling or debriefing to process difficult encounters.
- Celebrate small wins and moments of impact.
- Know when to rest, seek help, or step back.
-

Confidence and resilience are not fixed traits—they are practices. With support, reflection, and courage, nurses can strengthen their voice and sustain their advocacy for patients, teams, and themselves.

For practical advice on building resilience please see Appendix 11: Tips for Building Resilience

Conclusion

Advocacy is not an optional skill in nursing—it is a professional imperative. Whether you're protecting a patient's rights, challenging unsafe practices, or asserting your own boundaries, advocacy is how nurses, midwives, and health visitors uphold the values of safety, dignity, and equity.

This chapter has explored the realities of power dynamics in healthcare, the challenges of speaking up in multidisciplinary teams, and the importance of building confidence and resilience. These are not just communication skills—they are acts of leadership. They are how professionals protect what matters most, even when it's difficult.

Advocacy requires courage, clarity, and compassion. It also requires support—through supervision, peer networks, and reflective practice. When nurses advocate for others and themselves, they strengthen not only their teams but the entire healthcare system.

Your voice matters. Your insight matters. And your ability to speak up—especially when it's uncomfortable—is one of the most powerful tools you have. Advocacy is not just about changing outcomes—it's about changing culture.

Chapter 9: Reflective Practice and Growth

In nursing, growth doesn't just come from experience—it comes from reflection. The ability to pause, process, and learn from difficult conversations is what transforms everyday practice into professional development. Whether through supervision, journaling, or structured reflection, nurses, midwives, and health visitors can deepen their insight, strengthen their communication, and build emotional resilience.

Reflective practice is not a luxury—it's a necessity. It helps professionals make sense of complex interactions, navigate ethical dilemmas, and recover from emotionally charged moments. It also supports self-awareness, confidence, and continuous improvement.

This chapter explores how to use supervision and journaling as tools for reflection, how to learn from challenging conversations, and how to build a personal communication toolkit that supports clarity, compassion, and courage. Because when nurses reflect, they don't just grow—they lead.

Supervision

Using Supervision and Journaling

Reflective practice is most powerful when it's supported by structure. Supervision and journaling are two key tools that help nurses, midwives, and health visitors process difficult conversations, explore emotional responses, and grow professionally. They offer space to pause, think, and learn—turning experience into insight.

Supervision as a Reflective Space

Supervision—whether clinical, managerial, or reflective—is not just about oversight. It's a protected space for dialogue, emotional processing, and ethical exploration. In supervision, professionals can:

- Talk through challenging conversations or decisions.
- Receive feedback and validation.
- Explore emotional reactions and moral dilemmas.
- Identify patterns in communication and behaviour.

Supervision helps prevent burnout, supports resilience, and strengthens professional confidence. It's especially vital for lone workers, such as health visitors, who may face complex situations without immediate peer support.

Journaling for Clarity and Growth

Journaling is a simple yet powerful tool for reflection. It allows professionals to:

- Capture thoughts and emotions after difficult encounters.

- Identify triggers, patterns, and learning points.
- Explore values, boundaries, and communication styles.
- Track progress and personal development over time.

Journaling doesn't need to be lengthy or formal. Even a few lines after a shift can help clarify what happened, how it felt, and what could be done differently next time.

Examples of reflective prompts include:

- What stood out in today's conversations?
- How did I feel—and why?
- What did I learn about myself or others?
- What support do I need moving forward?

Integrating Reflection into Practice

To make supervision and journaling sustainable:

- Schedule regular supervision sessions and protect that time.
- Keep a dedicated journal or digital log for reflections.
- Use structured models (e.g., Gibbs, Schön, or Driscoll) to guide deeper thinking.
- Share insights with trusted colleagues or mentors when appropriate.

Reflection is not a sign of weakness—it's a sign of professionalism. It helps nurses stay emotionally attuned, ethically grounded, and communicatively confident.

Learning from Difficult Conversations

Difficult conversations are often uncomfortable—but they are also rich with learning. Whether the outcome was positive, unresolved, or emotionally charged, each interaction offers insight into communication, boundaries, and professional growth. Reflecting on these moments helps nurses, midwives, and health visitors refine their approach, strengthen their confidence, and deepen their emotional intelligence.

Why Reflection Matters

Without reflection, difficult conversations can linger as stress or self-doubt. With reflection, they become opportunities to:

- Understand what worked—and what didn't.
- Explore emotional responses and triggers.
- Identify communication strengths and areas for improvement.
- Reconnect with professional values and purpose.

Reflection transforms discomfort into development. It helps professionals move from reaction to response, and from confusion to clarity.

What to Reflect On

After a difficult conversation, consider:

- **The context**: What was the setting, and who was involved?
- **The emotions**: What did you feel before, during, and after?
- **The communication**: What language, tone, or body

language shaped the interaction?
- **The outcome**: What was resolved, and what remains unsettled?
- **The learning**: What would you do differently next time?

Using structured models like Gibbs' Reflective Cycle or Driscoll's "What?" model can help guide this process.

Turning Reflection into Action

Learning from difficult conversations means applying insights to future practice. This might include:

- Adjusting your communication style.
- Seeking supervision to explore unresolved emotions.
- Practising assertiveness or empathy in safer settings.
- Documenting key learning points in a reflective journal.

It also means recognising growth. Each difficult conversation you navigate adds to your skillset, resilience, and leadership capacity.

Building a Personal Communication Toolkit

Every nurse, midwife, and health visitor develop their own communication style—but intentional reflection can help shape that style into a reliable, adaptable toolkit. A personal communication toolkit is a set of strategies, phrases, frameworks, and self-awareness practices that support confident, compassionate dialogue across diverse situations.

Why a Toolkit Matters

In emotionally charged or ethically complex conversations, having a toolkit helps you:

- Stay grounded and focused.
- Respond with empathy and professionalism.
- Adapt to different contexts—hospital, community, home visits.
- Maintain boundaries while offering support.

It's not about having a script—it's about having options.

What to Include in Your Toolkit

Your toolkit might include:

- **Frameworks**: NURSE (for emotional distress), SBAR (for structured communication), SPIKES (for delivering difficult news).
- **Go-to phrases**: "Can you tell me more about that?" / "It's okay to feel overwhelmed." / "I want to make sure I

understand you correctly."

- **Body language awareness**: Open posture, gentle eye contact, calm tone.
- **Emotional regulation techniques**: Breathing exercises, grounding strategies, pause-and-reflect habits.
- **Reflective prompts**: Questions to ask yourself after a conversation—What went well? What felt difficult? What do I need?

Adapting Your Toolkit Over Time

Your communication toolkit should evolve with experience. Use supervision and journaling to:

- Identify what works well in practice.
- Explore moments of discomfort or uncertainty.
- Add new strategies based on learning and feedback.
- Remove habits that no longer serve you.

You might also tailor your toolkit to specific roles—e.g., safeguarding conversations, end-of-life care, or working with young people.

Toolkit as a Confidence Anchor

Having a personal toolkit builds confidence. It reminds you that you are prepared, supported, and capable—even in the most challenging conversations. It's a resource you carry with you, shaped by your values, your voice, and your commitment to compassionate care.

Conclusion

In healthcare, reflection is not a pause—it's a practice that sustains clarity, compassion, and confidence. It allows nurses, midwives, and health visitors to process emotional experiences, learn from difficult conversations, and grow with intention. Whether through supervision, journaling, or structured reflection, these tools help transform everyday challenges into meaningful professional development.

This chapter has shown that growth is not just about gaining experience—it's about making sense of it. Reflective practice deepens emotional intelligence, strengthens communication, and supports ethical clarity. It helps professionals stay connected to their values, adapt to complexity, and lead with empathy.

Your personal communication toolkit, shaped by reflection and experience, becomes a resource you carry into every interaction. It empowers you to speak with confidence, listen with compassion, and advocate with courage.

In a profession built on care, reflection is how we care for ourselves—and how we continue to care better for others.

Conclusion: Speaking Up, Growing Stronger

Throughout this book, we've explored the emotional, ethical, and professional dimensions of difficult conversations in nursing, midwifery, and health visiting. From navigating emotional distress and end-of-life care to addressing racism, safeguarding concerns, and team dynamics, each chapter has offered tools to help you speak up with confidence, compassion, and clarity.

You've learned how to:

- Use structured frameworks like NURSE, SBAR, and SPIKES to guide sensitive dialogue.
- Recognise and respond to emotional distress, microaggressions, and power imbalances.
- Advocate for patients and yourself in multidisciplinary teams.
- Reflect on challenging conversations through supervision and journaling.
- Build a personal communication toolkit tailored to your values and practice.

These strategies are not just for emergencies—they are for everyday care. They help you uphold professional standards, protect patient safety, and support your own wellbeing.

Ongoing Learning and Support

Difficult conversations are not one-off events—they are part of the ongoing relationship you build with patients, families, and colleagues.

As your career evolves, so will your communication style, emotional resilience, and ethical insight.

To continue growing:

- Engage in regular supervision and reflective practice.
- Seek out training in cultural competence, trauma-informed care, and inclusive communication.
- Connect with peer networks, mentors, and professional bodies for support and shared learning.
- Revisit this book as a toolkit—not just a guide—whenever you face a new challenge.

Resources for Further Support

To deepen your practice, consider exploring:

- **The Nursing and Midwifery Council (NMC) Code** – for professional standards and guidance.
- **Clinical and reflective supervision** – for emotional processing and ethical clarity.
- **Occupational health and counselling services** – for personal wellbeing.
- **Peer support groups and mentoring schemes** – for connection and shared growth.
- **Training platforms and CPD resources** – for ongoing skill development.

Final Reflection

Difficult conversations are not a sign of failure—they are a sign of leadership. They are how we protect patients, support colleagues, and uphold the values of our profession. When nurses speak up, care improves—and so do outcomes for everyone involved.

You already have the courage. This book has given you the tools. Now, keep growing, keep reflecting, and keep speaking up—because your voice matters.

Appendices

Appendix 1: Difficult Conversations in Nursing: Toolkit

Why Conversations Matter

- Avoidance leads to low morale, unresolved conflict, and compromised patient safety.
- Early intervention fosters psychological safety and team trust.
- Open dialogue supports inclusive, non-toxic work environments.

Barriers to Speaking Up

- Fear of emotional reactions or damaging relationships.
- Uncertainty about how to start or what to say.
- Lack of confidence, training, or support.
- Neurodiverse or cultural differences in communication styles.

Core Communication Skills

- Active listening: reflect feelings, clarify jargon, and use silence intentionally.
- Empathetic responses: validate emotions without judgment.
- Feedback: be factual, constructive, and solution focused.
- Questioning: use open questions to explore, closed to verify, reflective for depth.

Neurodiversity Considerations

- Adapt communication styles to support neurodiverse colleagues.

- Use clear, specific questions instead of open-ended ones when needed.
- Be mindful of sensory and emotional processing differences.

Structured Conversation Planning

- Before: Gather facts, check policies, choose a private space.
- During: Stay calm, listen actively, agree next steps.
- After: Document outcomes, follow up, seek supervision if needed.

Support Resources

- Clinical or reflective supervision.
- Occupational health and counselling services.
- Peer support groups and mentoring.
- Equality and diversity teams for neurodiversity guidance

Appendix 2: Conversation Frameworks Toolkit

Conversation Starters

- "You seem a bit quiet today—how are you feeling?"
- "It's okay to feel overwhelmed. Would you like to talk about it?"
- "I'm here to listen if there's anything you'd like to share."

Empathetic Responses

- "That sounds incredibly difficult."
- "It makes sense that you're feeling this way."
- "Thank you for trusting me with that."

Reflective Prompts for Practice

- What emotional cues did I notice today?
- How did I respond, and what impact did it have?
- What could I do differently next time?
- How am I feeling after that conversation—and what do I need?

Support Resources

- Clinical or reflective supervision
- Occupational health and counselling services
- Peer support groups or mentoring
- NMC Code and organisational policies

This toolkit is designed to be revisited regularly. Emotional conversations are not one-off events -they are part of the ongoing relationship nurses build with patients, families, and themselves. With practice, reflection, and support, these moments can become opportunities for healing, connection, and growth.

Appendix 3: End-of-Life Conversations: Toolkit

Conversation Starters

- "Would you like to talk about what's ahead?"
- "What matters most to you right now?"
- "Is there anything you'd like us to know about your wishes or values?"

Empathetic Responses

- "This must be incredibly difficult."
- "It's okay to feel uncertain or afraid."
- "Thank you for sharing that with me."

Reflective Prompts for Practice

- What emotional or existential cues did I notice today?
- How did I respond, and what impact did it have?
- What ethical dilemmas arose, and how did I navigate them?
- What support do I need after this conversation?

Support Resources

- Clinical or reflective supervision
- Palliative care and chaplaincy teams
- Occupational health and counselling services
- Ethics committees or senior clinical advisors
- Peer support groups or debriefing sessions

Appendix 4: Safeguarding Conversation Checklist

This checklist is designed to support nurses, midwives, and health visitors in initiating and managing safeguarding conversations with patients, families, and multidisciplinary teams. It includes key steps for preparation, communication, documentation, and follow-up.

Preparation:

- Review relevant safeguarding policies and procedures.
- Gather factual information and evidence before the conversation.
- Choose a private, safe, and appropriate setting for the discussion.
- Consider cultural, cognitive, and emotional factors that may affect communication.
- Seek advice from safeguarding leads or senior colleagues if needed.

Communication:

- Use plain, non-judgmental language to explain concerns.
- Be honest and transparent about the safeguarding process.
- Listen actively and validate emotions without blame.
- Use structured tools like SBAR to communicate risk clearly.
- Be prepared for emotional reactions and respond with empathy.

Documentation:

- Record concerns factually and objectively.
- Avoid assumptions or subjective language.
- Include dates, times, direct quotes, and observed behaviors.
- Document any actions taken and referrals made.

Follow-Up:

- Arrange follow-up meetings or check-ins as appropriate.
- Ensure referrals are actioned and outcomes monitored.
- Debrief with colleagues or supervisors to reflect on the conversation.
- Seek emotional support if the conversation was distressing.

Appendix 5: SBAR Template for Safeguarding Concerns

This template is designed to help nurses, midwives, and health visitors document safeguarding concerns using the SBAR framework. It provides a structured format for clear, concise, and professional communication when escalating concerns to safeguarding teams or multidisciplinary colleagues.

S – Situation

- What is happening now?
- Why are you concerned?
- Who is involved?

Example: 'I am concerned about Mrs. X, a 72-year-old patient who disclosed possible financial abuse by a relative.'

B – Background

- What is the relevant history?
- What do you know about the patient/family?
- Any previous safeguarding concerns?

Example: 'Mrs. X has a history of cognitive impairment and lives alone. She has previously declined social care support.'

A – Assessment

- What is your professional assessment?

- What risks have you identified?
- What is the impact on the individual?

Example: 'Based on her disclosure and presentation, I believe there is a risk of ongoing financial exploitation.'

R – Recommendation

- What do you recommend happens next?
- Who needs to be informed or involved?
- What support is required?

Example: 'I recommend an urgent referral to the adult safeguarding team and a review of her care plan.'

Appendix 6: Managing Workload and Burnout Toolkit

Self-Check Prompts:

- What tasks feel most draining—and why?
- When did I last feel joy or connection in my work?
- What support do I need right now?

Conversation Starters:

- *"I'm feeling overwhelmed—can we look at my caseload together?"*
- *"I'd like to schedule supervision to reflect on some recent challenges."*

Support Resources:

- Supervision and peer support groups
- Occupational health and counselling services
- Health passports and wellbeing plans
- NMC Code and employer policies on safe practice

Appendix 7: Leading Through Burnout Toolkit

Leadership Prompts:

- What support have I offered this week?
- Who might be struggling silently?
- How am I modelling emotional resilience?

Team Conversation Starters:

- *"Let's take a moment to check in—how's everyone doing?"*
- *"What's one thing that would make your week easier?"*

Support Resources:

- Reflective supervision and team debriefs
- Occupational health and wellbeing services
- Leadership development and coaching
- NMC guidance on professional support and accountability

Appendix 8: Raising Concerns Constructively Toolkit

Self-Check Prompts:

- What is the core issue—and what impact is it having?
- What support do I need to raise this safely?
- What outcome am I hoping for?

Support Resources:

- Supervision and reflective practice
- HR and whistleblowing policies
- Safeguarding leads and clinical governance teams
- NMC Code and professional guidance

Appendix 9: Peer Support and Supervision Toolkit

Self-Check Prompts:

- When did I last reflect on my emotional responses?
- Who do I feel safe talking to about work stress?
- What kind of supervision would support me best?

Conversation Starters:

- *"Could we schedule a reflective supervision session?"*
- *"Would you be open to a peer check-in this week?"*

Support Resources:

- Clinical, managerial, and reflective supervision
- Peer mentoring and buddy systems
- Occupational health and wellbeing services

NMC guidance on professional support

Appendix 9: Peer Support and Supervision Toolkit

Self-Check Prompts:

- When did I last reflect on my emotional responses?
- Who do I feel safe talking to about work stress?
- What kind of supervision would support me best?

Conversation Starters:

- *"Could we schedule a reflective supervision session?"*
- *"Would you be open to a peer check-in this week?"*

Support Resources:

- Clinical, managerial, and reflective supervision
- Peer mentoring and buddy systems
- Occupational health and wellbeing services

NMC guidance on professional support

Appendix 10: Allyship Toolkit for Nurses

Practical Strategies for Inclusive Practice in Healthcare Settings

Introduction

Allyship in healthcare is the active, ongoing practice of supporting colleagues who face discrimination or exclusion. For nurses, midwives, and health visitors, allyship is not about being a saviour—it's about standing in solidarity, amplifying marginalised voices, and challenging injustice. This toolkit summarises key strategies for fostering inclusive, respectful, and psychologically safe environments in diverse healthcare settings.

Allyship Strategies

- Speak Up Against Bias: Challenge discriminatory comments or behaviours respectfully. Use clear, assertive language to name the impact without blaming.
- Listen and Validate: Create space for colleagues to share experiences. Acknowledge emotions and avoid minimising or dismissing concerns.
- Educate Yourself: Learn about racism, privilege, and systemic inequality. Take responsibility for your own learning, don't rely on others to explain.
- Amplify Marginalised Voices: Support colleagues in meetings, projects, and leadership opportunities. Ensure diverse perspectives are heard and valued.
- Advocate for Inclusive Practices: Promote policies and training that support equity and belonging. Encourage inclusive recruitment, supervision, and team development.

- Reflect and Improve: Use supervision and reflective practice to examine your own biases. Be open to feedback and committed to growth.
- Build a Culture of Allyship: Model inclusive behaviour in everyday interactions. Support team norms that prioritise respect, safety, and accountability.

Closing Reflection

Allyship is not a one-off activity, it's a culture. When nurses act as allies, they don't just support individuals, they strengthen the entire team and improve care for all. This toolkit is designed to support ongoing reflection, dialogue, and action. Use it in training, supervision, and team development to foster environments where every voice is valued.

Appendix 11: Tips for Building Resilience

1. Practice Reflective Supervision

- Use structured models (e.g., Gibbs, Schön) to process emotional experiences.
- Reflect on what went well, what was challenging, and what you learned.

2. Develop Emotional Regulation Skills

- Use grounding techniques like deep breathing, mindfulness, or short breaks during shifts.
- Recognise emotional triggers and learn to pause before reacting.

3. Build Support Networks

- Connect with peers, mentors, or professional groups for validation and shared learning.
- Schedule regular check-ins or informal debriefs to reduce isolation.

4. Set Boundaries

- Learn to say no when needed and protect your time and energy.
- Separate work stress from personal life where possible.

5. Focus on Meaning and Purpose

- Reconnect with why you chose this profession.
- Celebrate small wins and moments of impact to reinforce your sense of value.

6. Use Self-Compassion

- Treat yourself with the same kindness you offer patients.
- Acknowledge that you're doing your best, even when outcomes are difficult.

7. Seek Help When Needed

- Access occupational health, counselling, or supervision if emotional distress affects your wellbeing.
- Asking for support is a strength, not a weakness.

8. Engage in Continuous Learning

- Build confidence through training, reading, and skill development.
- View challenges as opportunities for growth rather than threats.

Glossary

Emotional Distress

A state of emotional suffering often experienced by patients and healthcare professionals, marked by feelings such as anxiety, sadness, fear, or overwhelm. Recognising and responding to emotional distress is a key part of compassionate care.

Safeguarding

The process of protecting individuals—especially children and vulnerable adults—from abuse, neglect, and exploitation. Nurses have a legal and ethical duty to raise concerns and act to ensure safety.

Supervision

A structured professional relationship that provides support, reflection, and guidance. It helps nurses process emotional experiences, improve practice, and maintain wellbeing.

Reflective Practice

The process of thinking critically about one's experiences to learn and grow professionally. It involves examining actions, emotions, and outcomes to improve future practice.

Microaggressions

Subtle, often unintentional comments or behaviours that communicate bias or exclusion. These can undermine psychological safety and contribute to a culture of discrimination.

Allyship

The active and ongoing practice of supporting individuals who face discrimination or exclusion. It involves speaking up, listening, educating oneself, and advocating for inclusive practices.

Capacity

A person's ability to understand, retain, and weigh information to make an informed decision. Nurses assess capacity to ensure decisions are made ethically and legally.

Consent

Permission given voluntarily by a person with capacity, based on clear and understandable information. Valid consent is essential for ethical and legal healthcare practice.

Advocacy

The act of speaking up to protect the rights, wellbeing, and dignity of patients or oneself. Advocacy is a core nursing responsibility, especially in complex or hierarchical settings.

Resilience

The ability to recover from emotional challenges and adapt to stress. Building resilience helps nurses sustain compassionate care and protect their own wellbeing.

Communication Frameworks

Structured tools that guide sensitive conversations, such as NURSE, SBAR, and SPIKES. These frameworks support clarity, empathy, and professionalism in difficult interactions.

References

Introduction References

Charalambous, L. (2025). Approaching difficult conversations at work. *Primary Health Care, 35*(3), 12–13.

Edmondson, A. (1999). Psychological safety and learning behavior in work teams. *Administrative Science Quarterly, 44*(2), 350–383. https://doi.org/10.2307/2666999

Nursing and Midwifery Council. (2018). *The Code: Professional standards of practice and behaviour for nurses, midwives and nursing associates.* https://www.nmc.org.uk/standards/code/

RCNi. (2025). Conflict in healthcare: How to resolve issues calmly and safely [Podcast]. *RCNi Podcasts.* https://rcni.com/podcast-healthcare-conflict

West, M., & Dawson, J. (2012). *Employee engagement and NHS performance.* The King's Fund. https://www.kingsfund.org.uk/publications/employee-engagement-nhs-performance

Chapter 1 References

Bond, C. (2024). *Skills for communicating effectively with people who have mental health issues.* Nursing Standard, 39(12). Retrieved from https://shura.shu.ac.uk/34555

Hafskjold, L., Sundling, V., van Dulmen, S., & Eide, H. (2017). The use of supportive communication when responding to older people's emotional distress in home care: An observational study. *BMC Nursing, 16*(24). https://doi.org/10.1186/s12912-017-0220-8

Jin, T., Hong, S., Liu, J., Liu, L., Jia, S., & Shen, G. (2025). Emotion regulation strategy moderates the impact of emotional labor on burnout in psychiatric nurses: A cross-sectional study. *BMC Nursing, 24*, Article 687. https://doi.org/10.1186/s12912-025-03487-x

Nursing and Midwifery Council. (2018). *The Code: Professional standards of practice and behaviour for nurses, midwives and nursing associates*. Retrieved from https://www.nmc.org.uk/standards/code

RCNi. (2025). *Conflict in healthcare: How to resolve issues calmly and safely* [Podcast]. Retrieved from https://rcni.com/podcast-healthcare-conflict

USAHS. (2024). *The importance of effective communication in nursing.* University of St. Augustine for Health Sciences. Retrieved from https://www.usa.edu/blog/communication-in-nursing[1]

Nursing World. (2024). *Reflective practice in nursing: 4 key strategies.* American Nurses Association. Retrieved from https://www.nursingworld.org/content-hub/resources/nursing-leadership/reflective-practice-in-nursing[2]

Chapter 2 References

American Psychological Association. (2017). Resolution on palliative care and end-of-life issues. https://www.apa.org/about/policy/palliative-care-eol[3]

Baile, W. F., Buckman, R., Lenzi, R., Glober, G., Beale, E. A., & Kudelka, A. P. (2000). SPIKES—A six-step protocol for delivering

1. https://www.usa.edu/blog/communication-in-nursing/
2. https://www.nursingworld.org/content-hub/resources/nursing-leadership/reflective-practice-in-nursing/
3. https://www.apa.org/about/policy/palliative-care-eol%20

bad news: Application to the patient with cancer. *The Oncologist, 5*(4), 302–311. https://doi.org/10.1634/theoncologist.5-4-302[4]

Boston, P., Bruce, A., & Schreiber, R. (2011). Existential suffering in the palliative care setting: An integrated literature review. *Journal of Pain and Symptom Management, 41*(3), 604–618. https://doi.org/10.1016/j.jpainsymman.2010.05.010[5]

Isaacson, M. (2014). Clarifying concepts: Cultural humility or competency. *Journal of Professional Nursing, 30*(3), 251–258. https://doi.org/10.1016/j.profnurs.2013.09.011[6]

Livne, R. (2019). *Values at the end of life: The logic of palliative care.* Harvard University Press. https://doi.org/10.4159/9780674239869[7]

Chapter 3 References

Department of Health. (2005). *Mental Capacity Act 2005* (c. 9). London: The Stationery Office.

Department of Health and Social Care. (2014). *Care Act 2014.* London: The Stationery Office. Retrieved from https://www.legislation.gov.uk/ukpga/2014/23/contents

Gallagher, C., & Cross, C. (1990). Children Act 1989: An introduction. *Maladjustment & Therapeutic Education, 8*(3), 122–129.

Leonard, M., Graham, S., & Bonacum, D. (2004). The SBAR communication technique: Teaching a structured communication method. *Institute for Healthcare Improvement.* Retrieved from

4. https://doi.org/10.1634/theoncologist.5-4-302%20

5. https://doi.org/10.1016/j.jpainsymman.2010.05.010%20

6. https://doi.org/10.1016/j.profnurs.2013.09.011%20

7. https://doi.org/10.4159/9780674239869%20

https://www.ihi.org/library/tools/sbar-tool-situation-background-assessment-recommendation

Dung, N. T. (2020). Effectiveness of SBAR communication tool on patient safety: An integrative review. *Vinmec Times City International Hospital.* Retrieved from https://scholar.dlu.edu.vn/thuvienso/bitstream/DLU123456789/157306/1/CVv485V4S12021147.pdf

American Psychological Association. (2024). *Professional Practice Guidelines for Working with Adults with Complex Trauma Histories.* Retrieved from https://www.apa.org/practice/guidelines/adults-complex-trauma-histories.pdf

Northumbria University. (2023). Safeguarding vulnerable adults: The role of the registered nurse. *Research Portal.* Retrieved from https://researchportal.northumbria.ac.uk/en/publications/safeguarding-vulnerable-adults-the-role-of-the-registered-nurse

Chapter 4 References

Acas. (2014). *Challenging Conversations and How to Manage Them.* Advisory, Conciliation and Arbitration Service. Retrieved from www.acas.org.uk/publications

UHSussex NHS Foundation Trust. (2023). *Handling Difficult Conversations Toolkit.* Internal staff resource. Retrieved from www.uhsussex.nhs.uk

Nursing and Midwifery Council. (2018). *The Code: Professional Standards of Practice and Behaviour for Nurses, Midwives and Nursing Associates*. Retrieved from www.nmc.org.uk/standards/code

Health and Safety Executive. (n.d.). *Bullying at Work*. Retrieved from www.hse.gov.uk/stress/bullying.htm

CIPD. (2018). *Neurodiversity at Work.* Chartered Institute of Personnel and Development. Retrieved from www.cipd.org

Harvard Business Review. (2022). *The "Angry Black Woman" Stereotype at Work.* Retrieved from https://hbr.org/2022/01/the-angry-black-woman-stereotype-at-work

Chapter 5 References

Acas. (2014). *Challenging conversations and how to manage them.* Advisory, Conciliation and Arbitration Service. https://www.acas.org.uk/publications

British Journal of Nursing. (2025). *Understanding burnout in nurses: identification and coping strategies.* Retrieved from https://www.britishjournalofnursing.com[8] [1][9]

CIPD. (2018). *Neurodiversity at work.* Chartered Institute of Personnel and Development. https://www.cipd.org

Dall'Ora, C., Ball, J., Reinius, M., & Griffiths, P. (2020). *Burnout in nursing: a theoretical review.* Retrieved from https://nursing.jhu.edu[10] [2][11]

Healing Breaths. (2025). *Top Strategies to Prevent Burnout in Healthcare Workers.* Retrieved from https://healingbreaths.org[12] [3][13]

8. https://www.britishjournalofnursing.com/content/professional/understanding-burnout-in-nurses-identification-and-coping-strategies
9. https://www.britishjournalofnursing.com/content/professional/understanding-burnout-in-nurses-identification-and-coping-strategies
10. https://nursing.jhu.edu/wp-content/uploads/excellence/community/global-center/documents/research-articles/Burnout%20in%20nursing%20a%20theoretical%20review.pdf
11. https://nursing.jhu.edu/wp-content/uploads/excellence/community/global-center/documents/research-articles/Burnout%20in%20nursing%20a%20theoretical%20review.pdf
12. https://healingbreaths.org/blog/burnout-in-healthcare-workers/

Lind, Y. (2024). *5 Proven Strategies for Healthcare Leaders to Prevent Burnout and Boost Team Performance.* Retrieved from https://www.yashicalind.com[14] [4][15]

British Journal of Nursing. (2025). *The role of the nurse leader in facilitating effective support and communication to raise concerns.* Retrieved from https://www.britishjournalofnursing.com[16] [6][17]

HCPC. (2023). *Effective Clinical and Peer Supervision in the Workplace.* Retrieved from https://www.hcpc-uk.org[18]

Nursing and Midwifery Council. (2018). *The Code: Professional standards of practice and behaviour for nurses, midwives and nursing associates.* https://www.nmc.org.uk/standards/code

Peer Support Works. (2021). *National Practice Guidelines for Peer Specialists and Supervisors.* Retrieved from https://www.peersupportworks.org[19]

Royal College of Nursing. (2023). *Raising and Escalating Concerns: A Guide for Nurses.* Retrieved from https://www.rcn.org.uk[20]

---

13. https://healingbreaths.org/blog/burnout-in-healthcare-workers/
14. https://www.yashicalind.com/blog/prevent-burnout-boost-team-performance-healthcare-leaders
15. https://www.yashicalind.com/blog/prevent-burnout-boost-team-performance-healthcare-leaders
16. https://www.britishjournalofnursing.com/content/professional/the-role-of-the-nurse-leader-in-facilitating-effective-support-and-communication-to-raise-concerns
17. https://www.britishjournalofnursing.com/content/professional/the-role-of-the-nurse-leader-in-facilitating-effective-support-and-communication-to-raise-concerns
18. https://www.hcpc-uk.org/globalassets/resources/reports/research/effective-clinical-and-peer-supervision-report.pdf
19. https://www.peersupportworks.org/wp-content/uploads/2021/07/National-Practice-Guidelines-for-Peer-Specialists-and-Supervisors-1.pdf

SAMHSA. (2021). *Resources for the Supervision of Peer Workers.* Retrieved from https://www.samhsa.gov[21]

UHSussex NHS Foundation Trust. (2023). *Handling difficult conversations toolkit.* https://www.uhsussex.nhs.uk

Chapter 6: References

Care Quality Commission. (2025). *Regulation 20: Duty of candour.* https://www.cqc.org.uk/guidance-regulation/providers/regulations-service-providers-and-managers/health-social-care-act/regulation-20

Faubion, D. (n.d.). *15 excellent SBAR nursing examples + how to use it.* Nursing Process. https://www.nursingprocess.org/sbar-nursing-examples.html

Nursing and Midwifery Council. (2018). *The code: Professional standards of practice and behaviour for nurses, midwives and nursing associates.* https://www.nmc.org.uk/standards/code

Nursing and Midwifery Council. (n.d.). *Whistleblowing to the NMC.* https://www.nmc.org.uk/standards/guidance/raising-concerns-guidance-for-nurses-and-midwives/whistleblowing/

O'Donovan, R., & McAuliffe, E. (2020). A systematic review of factors that enable psychological safety in healthcare teams. *International Journal for Quality in Health Care, 32*(4), 240–250. https://doi.org/10.1093/intqhc/mzaa025

20. https://www.rcn.org.uk/-/media/Royal-College-Of-Nursing/Documents/Publications/2023/June/010-714.pdf

21. https://www.samhsa.gov/sites/default/files/programs_campaigns/brss_tacs/guidelines-peer-supervision-3-resources-cp4.pdf

Park, L. J. (2020). Using the SBAR handover tool. *British Journal of Nursing, 29*(14). https://www.britishjournalofnursing.com/content/clinical/using-the-sbar-handover-tool/

Chapter 7 References

Akbar, M. (2020). *Beyond ally: The pursuit of racial justice.* New Harbinger Publications.

American Psychological Association. (2020). *Publication manual of the American Psychological Association* (7th ed.). https://apastyle.apa.org

American Psychological Association. (2021). *Inclusive language guide.* https://www.apa.org/about/apa/equity-diversity-inclusion/language-guidelines

American Psychological Association. (2023). *Bias-free language guidelines.* https://apastyle.apa.org/style-grammar-guidelines/bias-free-language

Purdue Online Writing Lab. (n.d.). *APA stylistics: Avoiding bias.* Purdue University. https://owl.purdue.edu/owl/researchandcitation/apastyle/apaformattingandstyleguide/apastylisticsavoidingbias.html[22]

Tervalon, M., & Murray-García, J. (1998). Cultural humility versus cultural competence: A critical distinction in defining physician training outcomes in multicultural education. *Journal of Health Care for the Poor and Underserved*, 9(2), 117–125.

Sue, D. W., Capodilupo, C. M., Torino, G. C., Bucceri, J. M., Holder, A. M. B., Nadal, K. L., & Esquilin, M. (2007). Racial microaggressions in everyday life: Implications for clinical practice. *American*

22. https://owl.purdue.edu/owl/researchandcitation/apastyle/apaformattingandstyleguide/apastylisticsavoidingbias.html

Psychologist, 62(4), 271–286. https://doi.org/10.1037/0003-066X.62.4.271

Chapter 8 References

Advocating for Patients and Yourself, Kearns, E., Khurshid, Z., Anjara, S., De Brún, A., Rowan, B., & McAuliffe, E. (2021). Power dynamics in healthcare teams – a barrier to team effectiveness and patient safety: A systematic review. *BJS Open*, *5*(Supplement_1), zrab032.091. https://doi.org/10.1093/bjsopen/zrab032.091

McTighe, A. J., & Donovan, S. (2017). Group dynamics in healthcare settings: A strategic framework for cohesion. *Research in Psychology and Behavioral Sciences*, 5(1), 30–35. https://doi.org/10.12691/rpbs-5-1-5

Rogers, L., De Brún, A., & McAuliffe, E. (2023). Exploring healthcare staff narratives to gain an in-depth understanding of changing multidisciplinary team power dynamics during the COVID-19 pandemic. *BMC Health Services Research*, *23*, Article 419. https://doi.org/10.1186/s12913-023-09406-7

Akinlotan, O. (2024). Leading and managing a multidisciplinary team in health and social care: A critical and personal reflection. *British Journal of Nursing*, *33*(12). https://www.britishjournalofnursing.com/content/professional/leading-and-managing-a-multidisciplinary-team-in-health-and-social-care-a-critical-and-personal-reflection

Nursing and Midwifery Council. (2018). *The Code: Professional standards of practice and behaviour for nurses, midwives and nursing associates*. https://www.nmc.org.uk/standards/code/

Thompson, G., & Glasø, L. (2018). Situational leadership theory: A test from three perspectives. *Leadership & Organization Development*

Journal, 39(5), 574–591. https://doi.org/10.1108/LODJ-10-2017-0290

van Diggele, C., Bannon, S., & Ilic, D. (2020). Leadership and management in health care: A guide for students and professionals. *The Clinical Teacher, 17*(6), 625–629. https://doi.org/10.1111/tct.13200

Chapter 9 References

Gibbs, G. (1988). *Learning by doing: A guide to teaching and learning methods*. Further Education Unit.

Jasper, M. (2013). *Beginning reflective practice* (2nd ed.). Cengage Learning.

Rolfe, G., Freshwater, D., & Jasper, M. (2001). *Critical reflection for nursing and the helping professions: A user's guide.* Palgrave Macmillan.

Bultas, M. W., Taylor, J., Rubbelke, C., Schmuke, A. D., & Jackson, J. (2023). Anxiety and answer-changing behavior in nursing students. *Journal of Nursing Education, 62*(6), 351–354. https://doi.org/10.3928/01484834-20230418-01

Ryan, S. W., & Kramer, M. L. (2024). Nursing assessment, diagnosis, and planning. In B. J. Astle, W. Duggleby, P. A. Potter, P. A. Stockert, A. G. Perry, & A. Hall (Eds.), *Potter and Perry's Canadian fundamentals of nursing* (7th ed., pp. 186–211). Elsevier.

American Psychological Association. (2020). *Publication manual of the American Psychological Association* (7th ed.). https://apastyle.apa.org

Further Reading and Resources – Difficult Conversations in Nursing

The Nursing and Midwifery Council (NMC):

Provides professional standards, guidance on communication, safeguarding, and ethical practice. Visit: https://www.nmc.org.uk

Mind – Mental Health Support:

Offers resources on emotional resilience, burnout prevention, and wellbeing for healthcare professionals. Visit: https://www.mind.org.uk

Skills for Care – Communication and Supervision:

Provides training materials and guidance on reflective supervision, communication skills, and safeguarding. Visit: https://www.skillsforcare.org.uk

RCN (Royal College of Nursing) Learning Resources:

Includes toolkits, webinars, and articles on cultural competence, advocacy, and professional development. Visit: https://www.rcn.org.uk

Cultural Humility Toolkit – Stanford Medicine:

A practical guide for healthcare professionals to engage in culturally responsive care and communication. Visit: https://med.stanford.edu/diversity/toolkits/cultural-humility.html

Safeguarding Adults and Children – NHS England:

Official guidance and resources for safeguarding practice in healthcare settings. Visit: https://www.england.nhs.uk/safeguarding

Also by Rachael Benson

Difficult Conversations

Difficult Conversations in Nursing & Healthcare: A Practical Guide to Speaking Up with Confidence and Compassion

Difficult Conversations in Teaching and Education: A Practical Guide to Speaking Up with Confidence and Compassion

Domestic Abuse -Guidance for Professionals

Domestic Abuse Routine Enquiry

Safeguarding in Practice

Safeguarding in Practice: Working Together 2023 – A Guide for Multi-Agency Professionals

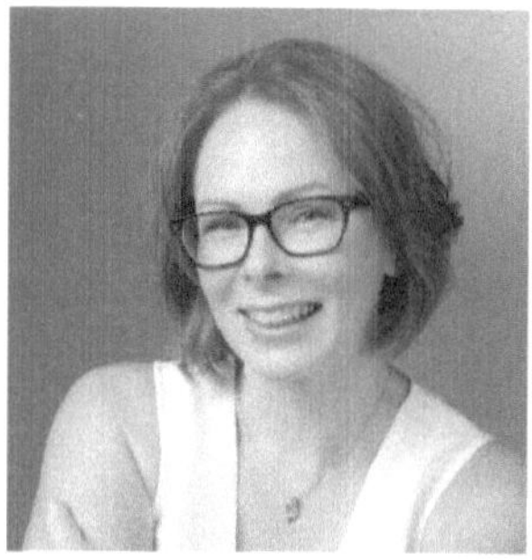

About the Author

Rachael Benson is a public health nurse, safeguarding consultant, and author with over two decades of experience supporting children, families, and professionals across health and social care. Specialising in early childhood development, emotional wellbeing, and safeguarding leadership, Rachael brings a compassionate, practical voice to the complex realities of frontline care.

She is the founder of **RCB SG Consultancy Ltd**, where she delivers training, supervision, and strategic guidance to organisations navigating safeguarding, burnout, and difficult conversations in healthcare. Her work is grounded in lived experience, evidence-based frameworks, and a deep commitment to equity, advocacy, and psychological safety.

Rachael's writing spans professional guides, wellbeing resources, and reflective tools for nurses, midwives, health visitors, and the multi-agency professional network. Her books empower readers to speak up with confidence, lead with integrity, and care with compassion—even in the most challenging moments.

When she's not writing or training, Rachael is developing innovative services for children and young people, mentoring professionals, and exploring the emotional dimensions of leadership and resilience.

www.ingramcontent.com/pod-product-compliance
Lightning Source LLC
LaVergne TN
LVHW090356210926
848480LV00002B/358